YOGA THERAPY
FOR
COMMON HEALTH PROBLEMS

(INCLUDING DRUG ABUSE, ALCOHOLISM & OBESITY)

Authors Choice Press
New York Lincoln Shanghai

To
My Wife
Shanti Devi

YOGA THERAPY FOR COMMON HEALTH PROBLEMS
(INCLUDING DRUG ABUSE, ALCOHOLISM & OBESITY)

Copyright © 1981, 2005 by PHULGENDA SINHA

Authors Choice Press
an imprint of iUniverse, Inc.

iUniverse books may be ordered through booksellers or by contacting:

iUniverse
2021 Pine Lake Road, Suite 100
Lincoln, NE 68512
www.iuniverse.com
1-800-Authors (1-800-288-4677)

Originally published by Yoga Institute of Washington, DC

Yogic Cure for Common Diseases
Copyright© 1976 by Phulgenda Sinha

First Printing: New Delhi, India, 1976

Second Printing: New Delhi, India, 1980

Revised and expanded edition
Yoga Therapy for Common Health Problems
Copyright© 1981 by Phulgenda Sinha.

ISBN-13: 978-0-595-36154-0
ISBN-10: 0-595-36154-4

Printed in the United States of America

Acknowledgement

I am greatly indebted to several of my students and friends for assisting me in various capacities in preparing the present revised edition of the book. I wish to express my heartfelt thanks to Betty Tihey for her painstaking work in editing and typing the complete manuscript and for her valuable suggestions. I must also thank Dr. Raymond Johnson for proofreading the whole manuscript and for his various noteworthy opinions and suggestions.

My indebtedness also extends to Charles M. Helmken for designing the cover and to Sean Mason for redrawing the sketches. I am indeed grateful to Dr. Vidyananda Singh, John Ficerai, Verne Myren, and Marco Carnivale for their encouragement, valuable advice, and help during the preparatory work on the manuscript.

Phulgenda Sinha

Washington, D.C.
June 1981

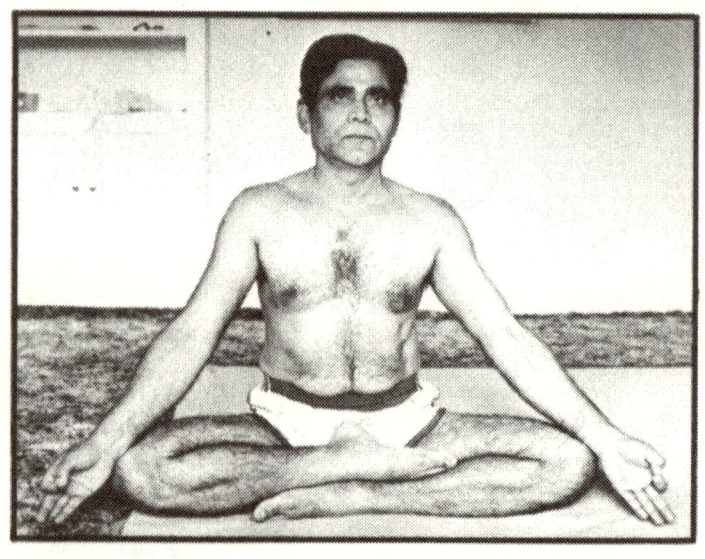

The Author in Siddha Asana

Preface

This book is the product of my years of experiences in treating patients of various diseases, disorders, and ailments through the yoga system. My experience at the Yoga Institute of Washington, D.C., from 1965 to 1968, and at the Indian Institute of Yoga, Patna, since 1969 has inspired me to write on Therapeutic Yoga.

The book, I am sure, will be a valuable contribution to the field of Therapeutic Yoga. Everything written, every *asana* prescribed, and all advice given in it are based on my research and personal experience while treating patients. The most significant feature of this book is that a person suffering from any of the health problems covered in it will have no difficulty in treating himself by following the guidelines described for the disease, along with the illustrations of yoga *asanas*.

Patients do not have to disturb their normal lives while practicing the prescribed *asanas*. Also, the diet in every case is almost normal. Though diet charts are provided for every disease, the general principles and methods of eating are the same as for any practitioner of yoga.

The *asanas*, *pranayamas*, and other *kriyas* recommended for a particular disease are such and so illustrated that a person of any physique can practice them easily. In the case of some difficult *asanas*, their easier forms are explained and illustrated together with the original ones.

It is very disheartening to note that a great majority of the books on Therapeutic Yoga make it compulsory for patients to do the *kriyas* of *Shat Karmas* (the six body purificatory processes) as a prerequisite for practicing Therapeutic Yoga. Most of the early books on yoga such as *Gherand Samhita, Goraksha Paddhati, Hatha Pradipika,* and *Vasistha Samhita* speak very highly of the benefits of these *Shat Karmas* and provide the details of practicing them. But it should be remembered that these *Shat Karmas* were primarily recommended for a few chosen *Sadhakas* (disciples) whose training in yoga was mainly for achieving spiritual, religious, and devotional ends. It should also be remembered that the *Sadhakas* who were asked to do the *Shat Karmas* were already in good health and practiced these techniques to purify themselves for gaining divine powers rather than being cured of diseases. Since most teachers of yoga therapy still recommend these practices to their patients and to the general public, let me enumerate these *Shat Karmas* and explain why they are not recommended to users of this book.

The *Shat Karmas* are the six purificatory techniques or processes. They are: *Dhauti, Basti, Neti, Trataka, Nauli,* and *Kapalbhati*. One major reason for not recommending them is that, unless done properly, they might cause grave injury and severe damage to practitioners. Those interested in learning any or all of these techniques must do so in the presence of a teacher and not with the help of any book, no matter how comprehensively written Because this book is written as a "guide for self-treatment," the practice of these purificatory processes is not advised.

In selecting the topics for this book, I have been faced with the problem of what to include and what to omit. Although I have treated several diseases and ailments such as tuberculosis, Parkinsonism, ulcers, polio, leucorrhoea, and impotence, they are not covered in this book. One major reason for excluding them is that the number of patients treated for these diseases was not enough to justify the claim of curing through Therapeutic Yoga as a proven system of treatment. Another is the size of this book. I have decided to cover only those diseases and disorders which are very common and of which I have long experience in treating.

With these considerations in mind, I shall cover (i) abdominal disorders, (ii) diabetes, (iii) asthma, (iv) arthritis, (v) obesity, (vi) mental problems, (vii) neck and spinal pain, (viii) sinus and headache, (ix) eye disorders, (x) heart ailments and high blood pressure, and (xi) alcoholism and drug abuse. These fifteen health problems are discussed in eleven chapters. The first chapter, which is basically an introduction, explains the value, method, and essentials of Therapeutic Yoga and offers a guideline for using a particular chapter to treat a particular disease. The last section provides a guideline for continuing yoga practice even after the particular ailments have been corrected.

For general practitioners of yoga also, this book will be very helpful and valuable. The methods of practicing *asanas*, *pranayamas,* and other *kriyas* are so clearly explained and illustrated that even beginners will have no difficulty in following them accurately. By selecting *asanas* according to the fitness of his body, any person can learn yoga with the help of this book.

Phulgenda Sinha

Table of Contents

List of Illustrations

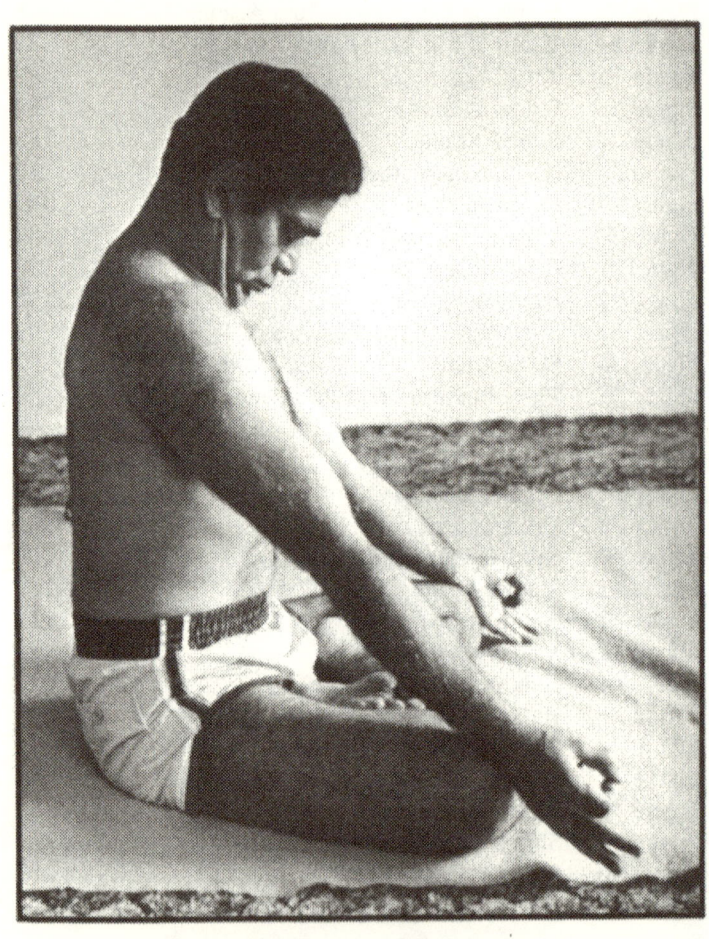

The Author in Jalandhar Bandha

CHAPTER 1

Therapeutic Yoga and Its Essentials

THERAPEUTIC YOGA is basically a system of self-treatment. According to yogic view, diseases, disorders, and ailments result from faulty ways of living: bad habits, lack of proper knowledge of things related to an individual's life, and an improper diet. The diseases thus result in a short or prolonged malfunctioning of the body's system. This malfunctioning is caused by an imbalanced internal condition, created by certain errors of individuals.

Since the root cause of a disease lies in the mistakes of the individual, its cure also lies in correcting those mistakes by the same person. This being the basic assumption in this system about the nature of the trouble and its remedy, there is a total reliance on the effort of the patient himself. The yoga expert shows only the path and works only as a counsellor to the patient.

The yogic process of treatment comprises three steps: (i) proper diet, (ii) proper yoga practice, and (iii) proper knowledge of those things which affect an individual's life. By following these steps, a disease can be cured.[1] A brief description of these steps is provided below:

Proper Diet: A diet is recommended according to the nature of the disease and the condition of the patient. The main idea about daily diet is to keep it balanced and to eliminate those items which are considered harmful in a particular disease. A diet chart for breakfast, lunch, afternoon refreshment, and dinner is prepared for each patient according to the condition of his body and the nature of his disease.

The most common dietary items for almost all patients of Therapeutic Yoga are fruits, salad, leafy and green vegetables, wheat bread, and selected legumes. For non-vegetarians, fish and liver are allowed in certain cases, but other kinds of meat, as well as chicken, are generally forbidden. Whatever the variations in the diet charts, patients are all asked to follow some basic principles of eating: eat slowly; eat only eighty-five percent of the stomach's capacity; eat at least two hours before retiring at night; avoid drinking water while eating; not to eat hot, spicy, and fried food; not to drink more than one or two cups of coffee or tea in a day or, if possible, to stop it completely; give up tobacco in any form; and avoid alcohol.

Yoga Practice: The patient should practice yoga according to his disease and his body's condition. In a majority of cases, a regular practice of only a few *asanas* is enough to cure the disease. In some diseases, the practice of *pranayama,* together with the *asanas,* is essential for good results. In certain cases, specific *kriyas,* such as *bandhas, mudras,* and certain yogic techniques, are used to produce the desired result. Besides these, the practice of concentration and meditation is also necessary in some instances.

In our research at the Indian Institute of Yoga at Patna, we

---

[1]The diseases referred to here are specially of the chronic type. We do not know yet if Yoga Therapy can cure all sorts of communicable diseases such as venereal diseases (V.D.), smallpox, and similar others, though even these can be prevented by yoga practice.

have found that a large number of diseases are cured within two months of yoga practice. In others, it takes about four months or even longer. Diseases that take a longer time are juvenile diabetes, polio, paralysis, Parkinsonism, ulcers, obesity, and mental illnesses.

It is interesting to note that the same *asanas, pranayamas, bandhas, mudras,* and other *kriyas* which are practiced for creative, preventive, and general health purposes are also used to cure diseases. But there is a difference in the manner of practice by a patient and that of the general practitioner. The patient with a particular disease is advised to do only as much of an *asana* as is possible for him.

By doing only what is physically performable, the patient gains strength as the *kriyas* begin to condition the body and diminish the illness. When the disease is cured, physical ability improves and the same *asanas* are performed even better by those who were unable to do them at the beginning.

Yoga therapy is a specialized form of yogic culture, and various yoga centers in India have developed their own systems based on their experience and research. In the absence of any standardization, there is some difference in the method of Therapeutic Yoga at various centers in India and elsewhere.[2]

Proper Knowledge: Though most patients are cured with only proper diet and yoga practice, some cases are more complicated. Some patients develop diseases and disorders because of their false assumptions; unhealthy habits; and lack of proper knowledge about life, nature, and society.

In such cases, many things which are informative, conceptual, and theoretical need to be explained to the patient. It is time-consuming work. Yogic literature is very rich in this respect and is divided into two main categories: spiritual and

---

[2]To understand this variation in Therapeutic Yoga, see the following sources: *Yoga Mimansa,* a quarterly journal of Kaivalyadhama, Lonavla (Poona); *Yoga,* a monthly journal of The Yoga Institute, Santa Cruz, Bombay; and *Yoga Science Journal,* a quarterly publication of the Indian Institute of Yoga, Patna.

scientific interpretations of things. However, the literature available in the second category is much less than that in the first one. Readers are best advised to have a scientific approach in all their reading on yoga.[3] Depending upon the nature of the disease, a patient is counseled and informed in detail about the various pertinent aspects of his life.

With this short description about the method of Therapeutic Yoga, it must be explained how it differs from the medical system of treatment.

Yoga vs. Medical System

In any medical system, the primary reliance is on medicine. It is assumed that a particular medicine will cure a particular disease. The medical doctor does the diagnosis, identifies the disease, and prescribes a suitable medicine. The patient in this system has to do very little or nothing at all; the task of correcting the disease or disorder and restoring the health is assigned to the medicine.

Seen in this context, there is a contrast between the medical and yoga systems of treatment. In the medical system an external agent (medicine) does the corrective work, while in the yoga system this external agent is not needed at all—it is the patient himself who, through his personal understanding, practice, and care, cures his own disease.

It would not be improper to mention that we have encountered several patients with chronic diseases who had lost their faith in the medical system because, despite years of treatment, they were not permanently and satisfactorily cured. In certain cases, the medicine gave them immediate relief, but not a lasting cure. On the other hand, many such patients were permanently cured through Therapeutic Yoga within two to four months. This has been especially so in cases of diabetes,

---

[3]Pertinent literature: Swami Vivekananda, *Jnana and Karma Yoga;* Kapil, *Samkhya Darshan;* Swami Sivananda, *Thought Power;* Swami Kuvalayananda, *Pranayama;* Yogendra, *Yoga Essays;* and Dr. Phulgenda Sinha, *Yoga: Meaning, Values and Practice.*

arthritis, asthma, gastrointestinal disorders, nervous tension, and various other conditions.

This limitation of the medical system should not imply that it is inferior to the yoga system; rather, it is only a matter of the limitation and scope of a given system. There are cases which only medical science and not yoga can cure. Similarly, there are certain diseases, which, though regarded as incurable by medicine, are definitely cured through yoga. This shows that every system of treatment has certain unique points as well as limitations.

Also, medical treatment has now become so expensive that millions of people all over the world cannot afford it. Yoga, on the other hand, does not involve any expenses.

Therefore, it would be prudent for medical men to adopt and use this tested and ancient system of yoga to treat those diseases and ailments whose medicinal cure is not certain. Since the system of Therapeutic Yoga has been scientifically established, it can be used as a "self-cure method" by people suffering from various disorders in any part of the world.

Essentials of Yoga Practice

People about to use this book as a guide for "self-treatment through yoga" must first be told about the suitability of time, place, body condition, dress, and other related matters. To derive the full benefit of Therapeutic Yoga, it is necessary to understand the following requirements and principles relevant to its practice:

Time: Although the morning, before breakfast, is regarded as best for practicing yoga, one can do it at any other time, provided the stomach is empty and not heavy with food. The general principle is to have an interval of three to four hours after eating and then do yoga. Also, there should be a gap of half an hour or so after drinking water, tea, or any juice. The body should be rested when practicing yoga.

The individual should select a time which is convenient for

his daily routine and should *try to do yoga at the same time every day.* A practice for at least five to six days a week should be enough to show improvement. Patients are advised to practice yoga only once in twenty-four hours unless specifically told to do so more often than that.

Place: Practice yoga on the floor. Use a carpet, rug, blanket, or mat on the floor. The place of practice should be neat, clean, and well ventilated. Windows should be kept open for cross ventilation. In summer, a fan can be used; but during winter, a cold draft should be avoided. If the place is air conditioned, make sure that there is a sufficient air supply.

Silence: One should maintain silence while doing yoga. There should be no conversation, mental activity, or even listening to music. Silence helps in preserving energy as well as in being attentive during practice.

Rest: There are two types of rest in yoga: the short and the long. The short rest, about six to eight seconds long, should be taken between two rounds of an *asana,* or between *asanas.* The shorter rest is done by breathing twice at the completion of one round of a posture.

The long rest comes at the end of all the *asanas, pranayamas,* and other *kriyas* which one does at a time. The general principle is to devote one-fourth of the actual practicing time for this rest. For example, if one has done yoga for twenty minutes, the rest at the end should be for five minutes.

This rest is done best in *Shava asana.* Those who cannot do *Shava asana* should just lie down on the floor, keep the eyes closed and the body loose, breathe normally, and concentrate on any place of natural beauty such as a garden, park, or hillside. In this simple method of resting, one should feel as if one were breathing the air of that chosen place and were relaxing by being mentally present there. After the rest is over, one should wait three to five minutes before eating or doing any work.

Dress: There should be a minimum of clothes on the body while doing yoga. Men can wear shorts or loose trousers and women can wear slacks or leotards. In winter, light woolen clothes may be worn.

Bath: People generally want to know whether a bath should be taken before or after yoga practice. For those practicing yoga in the morning, it is not necessary to bathe before. It depends on the convenience and personal choice of the practitioner whether to bathe before or after the practice. After yoga practice, one must wait for about fifteen minutes before taking a hot bath. Many people prefer to practice yoga after bathing because there are certain *asanas* which are done better then, and because the bath creates a feeling of neatness and purity.

Method of Practice: To obtain the fullest benefits of yoga, one must practice it properly. Since yoga is a scientific system, it must be done in a specified manner. If the *asanas, pranayamas, bandhas,* and *mudras* are not done according to the established methods, yoga will become merely an exercise and will not give satisfactory results. The benefit of yoga on the body is greater because ot its methodology.[4]

What is important to mention here is that, although everyone cannot practice all the postures perfectly, they can certainly follow the method of doing them without any difficulty. Therefore, do yoga according to the limitations of your body; do only as much as you can. You need not be perfect in forms. If you cannot do the full form, do half of it or even less.[5]

Follow all steps carefully. Also, it is important to begin the practice with only a few *asanas* during the first week. When two or three *asanas* have been practiced for a week, the next two *asanas* should be added during the second week. This way, new *asanas* can be added gradually every week, according to the need and recommendations in a given case.

---

[4]For understanding the scientific principles of yoga, see: Dr. Phulgenda Sinha, *Yoga: Meaning, Values and Practice* (Patna: Indian Institute of Yoga, 1970), pp. 2-8, or its

Female Problems: Women should not practice yoga during their menstrual periods or during advanced pregnancy (after the fourth month). Under such conditions, yoga practice should be generally discontinued. Yoga for pregnant women (after the fourth month) must be done on a selective basis under the proper care and instructions of the yoga expert.

It is significant to mention that yoga has a great curative value for various ailments and disorders of women. For example, menstrual disorders are corrected and normalized through yoga. The proper practice of yoga during the early stages of pregnancy enhances the health of the child in the womb and also helps to make the delivery painless.

How Much Yoga: Yoga can be practiced longer in the winter than in summer. The maximum time devoted for practice should not exceed forty-five minutes on a winter day. In summer, the maximum time for practice should be thirty minutes. This difference in practicing time has to be maintained because the weather has varied effects on the body.

Though there should be only one session of yoga practice in a day, those who would like to divide their time in two sessions should allow eight hours to elapse between the first and second sessions. A minimum practice of fifteen minutes per day should be quite satisfactory for maintaining good health.

With the above-mentioned clarifications about Therapeutic Yoga and its basic requirements, let us explain what is meant by "proper diet" in the yoga system. A proper understanding of some of the established principles and recommendations about diet will help practitioners to better realize the importance of food and its impact on the body. Though specific diet charts are given for different types of diseases, users of this book are advised to read the following section on "Proper Diet" for a more comprehensive knowledge of it.

---

paperback edition (Bombay: Jaico Publishing House, 1972), Chapter I.

[5]Those *asanas* whose final form cannot be performed with equal perfection by all, are mentioned with their variations in the text. In certain cases, the easier method and simple form of an *asana* are given.

Proper Diet

Diet is very important in the yoga system. It is said that "As you eat, so you become." This is because the kind and quality of food affect the physical as well as the mental condition of the individual. Thus, the individual who does not follow a proper diet, and who does not have a proper understanding of the principles of eating, gradually harms himself physically and mentally. He begins to feel the ill effects of wrong eating habits on his appearance, behavior, thought, and also on actions, which justifies the saying that "As you eat, so you become."

In yoga, all foods are divided into three categories: *Rajasi, Tamasi,* and *Sattvik.*

Rajasi: *Rajasi* food comprises a variety of dishes, and it derives its name from the dining manners of Indian kings. It is said that no less than fifty-six dishes were served at a royal dining table. Naturally, dishes of various kinds—some fried, some curried, and highly seasoned, together with different sweets and drinks—would be served. Foods of this type are regarded as undesirable for yoga practitioners because they add extra weight and fat, generate a feeling of heaviness for a long time after dinner, and arouse passion.

Tamasi: When any dish—vegetarian or non-vegetarian—is prepared with too many spices and with excessive salt, pepper, chili, and other such seasonings, it becomes *tamasi.* This type of food suits those who have a coarse nature and a rough temperament and who are inclined to be selfish, quarrelsome, and intolerant. Hence, this type of food is undesirable and not recommended to yoga practitioners.

Sattvik: In this type, food is cooked with the least amount of spices and without much seasoning. Though the food is fresh, attractive, and nutritive, it is cooked simply. This type of food is desirable and highly recommended for yoga practitioners.

According to yogic principles, no food, whether vegetarian

or non-vegetarian, is by itself *rajasi, tamasi,* or *sattvik.* What makes it this or that type is the method of preparation and not the food itself. The generally held notion that non-vegetarian food is *tamasi* and vegetarian food is *sattvik* is wrong, because potatoes or cauliflower can be prepared as *tamasi* and meat or chicken can be cooked as *sattvik,* depending upon the choice of the individual.

Another point which needs clarifying is that, in yoga, food is not evaluated on the basis of its caloric count. Rather, it is the quality of food and the method of eating it that are considered. The better the quality of food, the more invigorating it is considered. Many people wrongly believe that, by reducing the food intake or reducing calories, they would lose extra weight. Similarly, many others feel that they would gain weight by eating heavily. These notions are undesirable, because both extremes have a harmful effect on the individual. Whether a person is overweight or underweight, the yogic principles and methods of eating are the same. One can gain or lose weight without any ill effects on his health by following the same yogic method of eating. What then are the yogic principles of eating?

Balanced Diet

The most important principle is to eat a balanced diet. When the following four things are included in the daily diet, it becomes balanced. These items are: salad, fresh vegetables, fresh fruits, and raw nuts. Whether you are a vegetarian or non-vegetarian, include these four items with your major dishes of the day.

Salad: All vegetables that are eaten raw constitute salad. Cucumbers, tomatoes, carrots, lettuce, cauliflower, etc., are used for salad. These should be cut into pieces and, with a little dressing, can be eaten raw in the quantity of about a cup per day. The ideal time to eat salad is to make it the first course of lunch and dinner.

Fresh Vegetables: Any vegetable which is not dried and not deformed is regarded as "fresh." They should be as fresh as possible. Fresh vegetables, whether from under or above the ground, must be eaten in a proportion to the other items taken during the meal. They should, of course, be prepared in a *sattvik* way.

Fresh Fruits: Fruits are the most nutritive food for any individual. For best results from yogic practice, fresh fruits are essential. It is not necessary that one eat only costly fruits; any that are easily available would serve the purpose. Fruits can be eaten alone or mixed with others. They may be seasonal or those available year-round. How much to take? One apple, one orange, or one banana a day, for example, would be enough for an individual. The important point is that fruits should be eaten regularly for better health.

Raw Nuts: Those nuts which are taken from hard shells are recommended and include cashews, pistachios, almonds, pecans, and walnuts. A handful mixture of these nuts is sufficient for a day. Since raw nuts have a warming effect on the body, they should be eaten in the winter and avoided or taken less in summer. Nuts from hard shells are full of proteins, minerals, and vitamins. Therefore, a proper intake of them is very energizing and healthy for the yoga practitioners and non-practitioners alike.

Besides the above-mentioned items of balanced diet, other principles of diet must be followed for satisfactory results. They are:

Quantity of Food

Eat no more than about eighty-five percent of your stomach's capacity. When food is taken in less than one's full capacity, it is easily digested and the body makes better use of it. But, when food is taken excessively and the stomach is completely stuffed, the food is not properly digested and the body is forced to eliminate it without making proper use of it. Further, by eating more, an individual overstrains the abdominal system in particular and the body in general, and his physical and mental powers become obstructed. The natural outcome of overeating is extra and unnecessary weight.

Method of Eating

The proper method is to eat slowly and swallow the food after thoroughly crushing and chewing it. One common mistake which overweight people generally make is that they all eat too fast. To them, chewing and then swallowing is perhaps unnecessary and boring. I recall a news item about a Texan whose dinner consisted of 18 chickens. He weighed more than 500 pounds, and he could not do much physical work. If he paid due attention to chewing all the chickens properly, he would be spending at least six to eight hours a day just for dinner, not including his breakfast, lunch, and other refreshments. The repercussions of this type of eating have already been explained.

The yogic system, thus, considers the ill effects of fast eating and emphasizes the importance of eating slowly. But the question is: How slow? It depends on the type of food one is eating. For example, a banana can be chewed faster than an apple. Eating meat would take more time than fish. But, in all circumstances, the guideline is to chew the food thoroughly and only then swallow it.

There are many benefits to eating slowly. The individual gets full satisfaction even when he eats only a small quantity of food. Saliva can be properly mixed with the food and makes it easier to digest. The body makes full use of any food taken and the individual maintains better health by consuming less.

Time Factor: Eat at least two hours before retiring. A common error with most people is that they eat and then soon go to sleep, especially at night. This is very harmful to their health. By eating hours ahead of sleeping, the food is properly processed by the body. The stomach is not heavy and, when the individual goes to bed, he gets undisturbed sleep and rest. Most people who complain of abdominal, stomach, or bowel troubles are in the habit of eating and then immediately going to sleep. By doing so, they put undue strain on the abdominal muscles; they get disturbed sleep; and, most of the time, they suffer from digestion ailments and disorders. Attention and care for eating early would correct these problems.

Another important point which needs clarifying is how many times one should eat. One should eat four times in twenty-four hours. This means having breakfast in the morning, lunch at noon, some refreshment in the afternoon, and dinner in the evening. The individual should eat according to his choice and preference, while keeping in mind the yogic principles. Except for special occasions, eating four times daily should become a habit.

Spices: It is recommended that not too much spice be used when preparing various dishes. This means not using too much salt, chili, peppers, and other herbs. Seasoning can be done for flavor, but excessive use should be avoided. Food should be seasoned so that it does not become *tamasi*, but remains *sattvik* in nature.

Water: It is recommended that yoga practitioners drink about ten to twelve glasses of water every day. Water should not be taken while eating, but half an hour later. According to yogic literature, several skin diseases and disorders are corrected if water is not taken while eating. Drinking plenty of water is highly recommended in yogic literature, because it is held that water cleans and washes out the impurities in the system. Many people do not drink enough water. I have known some people who were in the habit of drinking very little or no water at all. Instead, they would drink juice, milk, and other liquids. As a result, they developed numerous ailments and physical disorders. But most of these ailments were corrected when they started drinking plenty of water daily. Therefore, yoga practitioners should drink the recommended amount of fresh water within twenty-four hours.

Coffee and Tea: Both coffee and tea are injurious to health when taken in excess. People are so used to tea and coffee in their daily lives that it is not easy to discontinue them. But their intake must be limited to maintain better health. No more than two cups of tea or coffee should be taken in twenty-four hours, because both these drinks, if taken in large quantities, cause constipation, insomnia, nervous tension, and other internal disorders. It has also been felt that an excess of these beverages distorts the natural complexion of the skin and roughens the facial tissues.

Alcoholic Drinks: All alcoholic drinks are regarded as vitamin thieves; they steal and destroy the nutrients of the system. Our objection to alcoholic drinks is not that they are intoxicants, but mainly because they weaken the individual, physically and mentally, if taken without restraint. The destructive power of alcoholic drinks is greater in hard liquors and lesser in weaker ones. But, regardless of the high- or low-alcoholic percentage, if drinking is a daily habit, it would prove extremely harmful. Therefore, yoga practitioners should avoid drinking alcohol everyday.

Gram (chick-peas): Sprouted gram (chick-peas) is a very nutritious grain. It is full of proteins, minerals, and vitamins. A regular intake of a handful of germinated gram is highly conducive to good health. Yoga practitioners are, therefore, advised to make it a part of their daily diet. Green grams can be eaten fresh. The ripe ones should be eaten after soaking them in water for about eight hours. Sprouted grams are better than the plain ones because they are enriched with energy derived from the air and light. (If a person cannot eat raw nuts and fruits regularly, he can compensate for this loss by eating sprouted grams instead.)

The recommendations on diet can be summed up by saying

that yogic dietary principles are so simple that yoga practitioners (whether vegetarian or non-vegetarian) should have no difficulty in following them. If these principles are followed closely and if the individual makes a habit of eating according to these recommendations, he will maintain good health. A good balanced diet, along with proper hygienic care and a regular practice of yoga, guarantees developing and maintaining a proportionate figure and dynamic health.

Bathing and Cleaning

Water is one of the three important things for human survival. The other two are air and food. Hence, a discussion about the value and uses of water is necessary. We know that several plants flourish only on water and that some people can survive on water alone for weeks and even months. This proves that there are life-nourishing elements in water. This being the importance of water, yoga practitioners must make proper use of it by taking sufficient water.

Water can be used internally and externally. In the preceding pages, where we recommended drinking at least ten glasses of water within twenty-four hours, the use is internal. Its external use is through washing and bathing.

In summer, one can bathe twice daily. In winter and other seasons, bathing once a day is necessary to maintain good health. One can use hot or cold water for bathing, according to personal preference and weather conditions.

How this external use of water benefits the individual should be explained. For this, we must understand the structural and functional aspects of *romekoops* (pores).

The word *romekoop* is made up of two Sanskrit words (*rome* + *koop*). *Rome* means "hair" and *koop* means "well." Thus, its literal meaning would be a hair-well, which is called a "pore" in English. We have millions of hairs on our bodies and the root of each hair goes deeper in the body from the upper layer of the skin. At the root of every hair is a tiny hole which is not visible to the naked eye; these tiny holes are called *romekoops*.

The body discards sweat and impurities of the system through these *romekoops* and allows air and water to penetrate through them.

Hence, the primary consideration is how to make good use of the pores for benefiting the system. This is achieved by rubbing the whole body thoroughly while bathing, as it serves several purposes in a single process. But how to rub and how to clean?

Rubbing: There are several ways of rubbing the body during the bath: with the palms, washcloth, sponge, or brush. But the best thing to rub the body with is a washcloth or small towel. Soak the washcloth in water, apply some soap to it, and rub the whole body with it firmly while bathing. This rubbing opens the pores, exercises the upper layers of the skin, and makes it possible for the body to receive energy and life-nourishing elements by soaking in the water. This rubbing can be done with or without soap. After rubbing the body, plenty of fresh water should be poured on it.

Body Cleaning: Since we are talking about the bath, it is also necessary to discuss soaps. In our times, it is very difficult to think about taking a bath without soap. Though we are not opposed to using soap, it must be understood that there are certain chemicals in it which do not suit the nature of the skin of every individual. As we know, many people get rashes and rough skin after using certain soaps. Also, except for cleaning the body, soaps do not contribute much to the good of the body. Thus, if you must use soap, select one of good quality which is agreeable to your skin.

In the yogic system, the method of cleaning is different. There are several substitutes for soap which not only clean the body but also contribute potentially to its health.

One good substitute for soap is gram (chick-pea) flour. Take a handful or more of gram flour and make a paste of it with lukewarm water in a cup. Before bathing, rub this paste over the whole body with the palms. After rubbing, wash the body with hot or cold water. The body will be cleaner than if soap had been used and it will become smooth, soft, and invigorated with energy.

We have already said that grams contain minerals, proteins, and vitamins. Thus by using gram flour, the bather receives two benefits at once—cleaning as well as invigorating the body. Also, gram flour cures many skin diseases and troubles such as itching, rough skin, and other similar disorders.

It is recommended that gram flour be used at intervals of two to three days. This flour can also be used for cleaning the face and for shampooing. Though the process for cleaning the face is the same as for cleaning the body, some extra work is involved in shampooing the hair.

Shampooing: Take the kneaded flour and make a paste of it. Then put it in a thin cloth and tie it up. Now squeeze that "paste-containing cloth" in water until the soft part is mixed with the water and only the rudiments remain in the cloth. When the paste has been well squeezed in water, throw the rudiments away and use that liquid-type paste for shampooing. The filtered paste will clean the hair in a very satisfactory and healthy way. Those who prefer to use other types of shampoos should choose them carefully. The hair should be shampooed once or at most twice a week.

Hair: Hair is the index of the health of the individual. Healthy hair generally means a healthy person. One simple way to keep the hair healthy is to rub at its roots when bathing. The process is to put some water on the head and rub the roots of the hair with the fingertips until a warming effect is felt. After rubbing for a minute or so, pour plenty of water on the head. After the bath is over, dry the head with a clean and dry towel. Then, if one prefers to use it, apply hair oil and comb the hair. Comb the hair twice or three times a day by giving a pull of the opposite, i.e., from the top down, from down up, left to right, and right to left. By this combing, the hair will be stronger and would be prevented from falling out.

Some people falsely believe that, by rubbing and combing,

they will lose their hair. Though a person who has dandruff might lose some hair by rubbing and combing in the initial stage, the hair would stop falling out after a week or so. Moreover, new hair would soon begin to grow. This rubbing and combing method is equally good for men and women.

Teeth: Like hair, teeth also symbolize the health of an individual. The simple way of keeping the teeth healthy is to brush them and massage the gums. Besides the morning cleaning, teeth must be brushed before retiring at night.

Brushing should be done in upward and downward motions and not sideways. Next, rub both sides of the gums firmly. It is sufficient to rub the gums with paste or toothpowder once in twenty-four hours. This makes the gums stronger and stops decay.

Oil Massage: Among the various oils used for massaging, mustard oil is the best. Mustard oil is very commonly used in India for cooking, applying to the hair, etc. It is also used to massage babies, as well as by wrestlers and old people. It is a healthy and invigorating oil. Since it has a warming effect on the body, yoga practitioners are advised to apply it only during winter and not during summer. When it is applied to the body, it penetrates through the pores and imparts elasticity and strength to the muscles, bones, and nerves. It soothes, cleans, gives a good tanned complexion to the body, and makes the skin healthy. It also helps to remove wrinkles and dry skin.

How should it be used: Take some oil on the palms, smear it on parts of the body, and lightly rub until the oil has partially soaked into the body. Then apply it all over the rest of the body and leave it there for about ten to fifteen minutes. In that time, part of the oil will be absorbed by the body through the pores.

You can clean the oil from the body in two ways. One is to shower without using soap and rub the body with either warm or cold water. Afterwards, wipe the oily remnants from the body with a dry clean towel. As the oil is wiped off, the body will gain a clean and smooth look.

The second process is that, after you have applied the oil, use gram-flour paste as a substitute for soap. Apply the paste all over the oily body and rub it with the palms until the paste is fully mixed with the oil. After this is done, wash off the mixture with either cold or hot water. Gram-flour paste will remove the oil more thoroughly and satisfactorily than soap can. By so doing, you benefit from both the oil and flour. This can be regarded as a beautifying treatment, as it enhances the natural look of the skin.

This application of oil and cleaning with the paste should be done on alternate days, or once or twice a week, but not everyday. If one prefers to use soap between the applications of oil and paste, there is no objection. If soap is used, it should be one that is agreeable to the nature and condition of the skin of the user.

Let me sum up this chapter by saying that all the basic information and suggestions regarding Therapeutic Yoga have been carefully outlined in the foregoing pages. You are advised to thoroughly read this whole chapter first so that you properly understand this yogic system of treatment before starting the actual practice. Remember that you are following "a system of self-treatment" without relying on or using medicine. Therefore, it is important that you understand it first for a satisfactory result. Keeping in mind the contents of this chapter, choose the section of your concern and begin the practice of yoga according to the guidelines given.

CHAPTER 2

Abdominal Disorders

ALL troubles that disturb the normal functioning of the digestive system are termed here as abdominal disorders. The most common ones are: constipation, wind formation, indigestion, dysentery, diarrhea, acidity, stomachache, and various forms of gastrointestinal disorders. Our experience shows that abdominal problems are widely prevalent, affecting young and old alike.

The most common causes of abdominal disorders are: (i) psychosomatic factors such as nervousness, tension, and various forms of stress and strain; and (ii) improper eating habits such as overeating, eating at irregular hours, an imbalanced diet, excessive use of hot spices and fried foods, eating adulterated and stale foods, not chewing food properly, or unhygienic eating habits.

We have found that these disorders are easily cured through the yoga system of treatment. In most cases, the ailment is controlled within two weeks and fully cured in about two months. Those suffering from these troubles can cure themselves by following the yoga system of practice.

The yoga system of treatment requires proper diet and the daily practice of a few *asanas*. Mention of some important points about proper diet must be made before the diet chart is described.

Proper Diet: Eat a balanced diet, which includes salad, green vegetables, and fresh fruits, along with other dishes of the day. Eat at least two hours before going to bed at night, and never eat more than about eighty-five percent of your stomach's capacity. Do not drink water during meals, but only after about half an hour of finishing your meals. Take ten to twelve glasses of water every day. Avoid fried and spicy foods. Exclude red pepper, pickles, and chutney from your daily menu. Do not drink more than two cups of tea or coffee in a day; if possible, stop taking tea and coffee for a while. Also, do not take carbonated beverages. Stop drinking tea or water upon arising in the morning. Non-vegetarians can eat fish or liver, but should avoid other meats for a while. People with any abdominal disorder should follow the diet chart given below:

Breakfast (7 to 9 A.M.)

(*i*) Any fruit or vegetable juice	—	one cup
(*ii*) Fresh apple or any other fresh fruit	—	as desired
(*iii*) Sprouted chick-peas	—	handful
(*iv*) Whole wheat bread	—	one or two slices
(*v*) Cheese	—	one slice
(*vi*) Egg (boiled or poached)	—	one
(*vii*) Herb tea, decaffeinated coffee, or Ovaltine	—	one cup, if desired

Lunch & Dinner (12 to 2 P.M.; 6 to 8 P.M.)

(*i*) Salad (a mixture of lettuce, carrot,

tomato, radish, cucumber, celery,
watercress) with salt, pepper, and — medium
lemon juice, or with salad dressing bowl

- (ii) Vegetable or bean soup — one cup
- (iii) Rice or whole wheat bread — as desired
- (iv) Green vegetables (any kind) — one cup
- (v) Leafy vegetables (spinach, broccoli,
  turnip or collard greens) — as desired
- (vi) Yogurt, cottage cheese, or buttermilk — if desired,
  in a small
  quantity

Afternoon Refreshments (3 to 4 P.M.)

- (i) Fresh fruit — any type
- (ii) Crackers — one or two
- (iii) Cheese — one slice
- (iv) Herb tea, decaffeinated coffee, — one cup,
  or Ovaltine if preferred

Yoga Practice: The important *pranayama* and *asanas* for correcting abdominal disorders are: *Pranayama* with *Rechaka* and *Puraka*, *Uttanapada asana*, *Pawana Mukta asana*, *Bhujanga asana*, *Shalabha asana*, *Pashchimottan asana*, and *Shava asana*. The methods of practicing these *asanas* and *pranayama* are described and illustrated in the following pages.

PRANAYAMA (with Rechaka and Puraka)

Pranayama is a special kind of breathing exercise. There are various forms of *pranayama;* though each is done differently, most have these three steps in common:

Rechaka (Exhalation)
Puraka (Inhalation)
Kumbhaka (Retention)

In this particular *pranayama*, there are only *rechaka* and *puraka* but no *kumbhaka* (retention of the breath). One significant aspect of this *pranayama* is that it is a diaphragmatic breathing. In this exercise, the stomach is rhythmically pulled in and out. It is very important to remember that the stomach is not pushed upward and downward.

Position of Readiness: Sit on the floor either in the *Padma asana* (Lotus pose), as shown in Figure 1, or in the *Sukha*

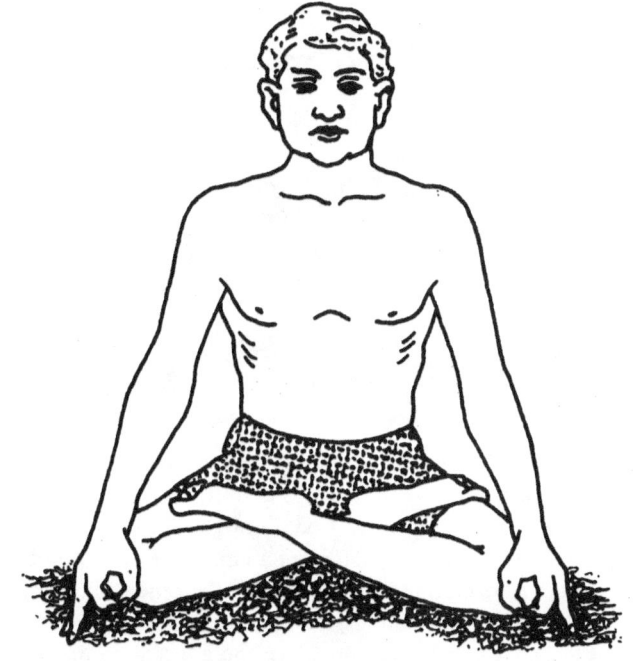

Figure 1. Padma Asana

asana (Easy pose), as shown in Figure 2.

To perform the *Padma asana*, stretch out your legs in front. Bend the right leg at the knee and bring the right foot (by lifting it slowly with the hands) onto the left thigh.

Then bend the left leg at the knee and place this foot on the right thigh. Both knees should touch the floor or should be as

35

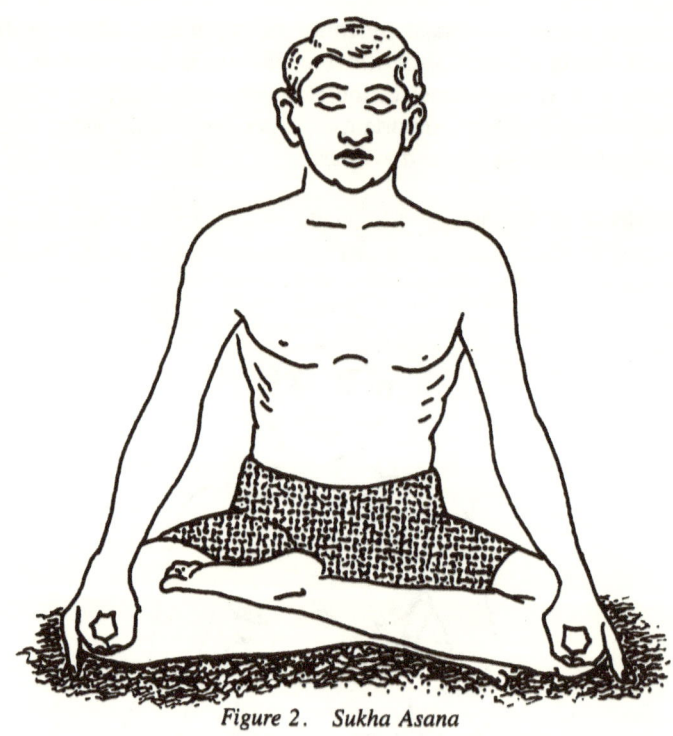

Figure 2.   Sukha Asana

near to it as possible. *Do not* exert pressure to lower the knees; they will gradually fall on the floor by themselves. *Keep the spine, neck, and head erect*. Look straight ahead at eye level. Place the wrists on the knees. Form a circle with the thumb and index finger of each hand and straighten the other three fingers, keeping them together and pointing downwards. Let the wrists rest on the knees. Breathe normally. You are now in the perfect position of *Padma asana*. Those who cannot sit in the *Padma asana* should sit in the *Sukha asana*.

To perform the *Sukha asana*, stretch out both legs in front. Bend your right leg at the knee and bring the sole of the right foot near the left thigh and place it on the floor. Your right knee should rest on the floor.

Then bend the left leg at the knee, lift it by hand, and place it on top of your right leg. Your left foot is now resting on the right foot and your left knee is a little above ground level.

Now straighten the spine, neck, and head in one line and make a circle with the thumb and the index finger as done for the *Padma asana*.

Note: Except for the difference in crossing the legs, other things are the same in both forms.

Steps of Actual Practice: (i) Exhale slowly through the nostrils and simultaneously pull your stomach inwards, i.e., contract the abdominal muscles to expel the air from your lungs. Keep exhaling until all the air is expelled.

(ii) Having exhaled, remain in this position for a second and then slowly start inhaling through both nostrils. Inhale as deeply as you can by stretching out the abdominal muscles. The expansion of the stomach should be gradual and rhythmic, not abrupt and fast.

(iii) After inhaling deeply, pause for a second and then start exhaling again. Repeat this process ten to fifteen times (one exhalation and one inhalation each time).

Daily Practice: During the first week, do this exercise ten times daily. During the second week and afterwards, increase it to fifteen times. Do not do it more than fifteen times in a single day.

Special Attention: When performing this *pranayama*, it is essential to keep the head, neck, and spine in a straight line. After the exercise is over, remain in the same position for a few seconds and breathe normally. Then gradually relax into a more comfortable position. Do other *asanas* after waiting for five to ten seconds.

Benefits: This *pranayama* activates all the organs of the digestive system. Because of this internal activation, problems such as constipation, dysentery, diarrhea, gastritis, indigestion, and stomachache are corrected.

This *pranayama* also affects various endocrine glands. The adrenal glands, pancreas, ovaries in women, and testicles in men are specifically activated and energized. Because they are activated, these glands begin to normally secrete their respective hormones.

Disorders of the circulatory and respiratory systems are also corrected. It is an easy *pranayama* and can be practiced without any difficulty by anyone.

UTTANAPADA ASANA
(LIFTING LEGS POSE)

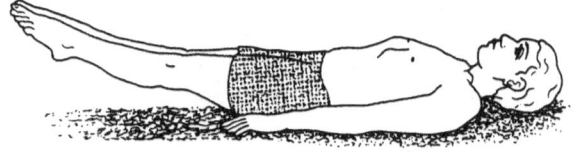

Figure 3.   Uttanapada Asana

Position of Readiness: Lie with your back on the floor and look towards the ceiling. Keep both arms straight alongside the body with the palms touching the floor. Straighten both legs and keep the heels and toes together. Breathe normally.

Steps of Actual Practice: (i) Inhale slowly but deeply through both nostrils and hold the breath.

(ii) Point the toes as much as you can.

(iii) Slowly lift both legs about ten to twelve inches from the floor and keep them there for six to eight seconds while holding the breath (Figure 3).

(iv) Then slowly start exhaling and lowering the legs, synchronizing both acts so that the legs reach the floor as you finish exhaling.

(v) Rest for two normal breaths, which should take about five to six seconds.

(vi) After resting, repeat the process.

Daily Practice: Four times daily. Do not practice more than five times in a single day.

Note: Those who have ever had any back injury or are otherwise weak should not do this *asana* with both legs. They should practice *Uttanapada asana* with one leg at a time until they get used to its impact (Figure 4). After practicing with one leg at a time for about four weeks, practice with both legs together.

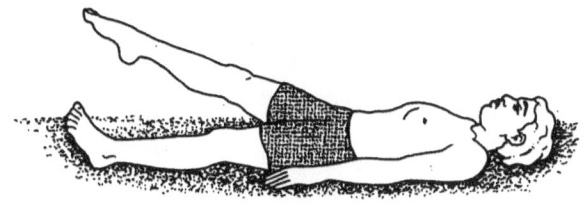

Figure 4.   Uttanapada Asana With One Leg

The reason for this precaution is that *Uttanapada asana* greatly strains the whole spine, as well as the rest of the body. This strain is cut in half by doing the *asana* with one leg only. The process of doing it with one leg is the same as for doing it with both. The only difference is that, instead of lifting both legs together, you lift only one leg and leave the other on the floor. Do it alternately, completing three times with each leg. Do not practice for more than six times at a stretch.

Benefits: The *Uttanapada asana* exercises all the abdominal muscles internally and externally. As a result, it corrects disorders of the pancreas and cures constipation, wind troubles, indigestion, and intestinal disorders. It eliminates extra weight of the abdominal area.

This *asana* also corrects backache or troubles in the waist, buttocks, and hip joints. It strengthens the spinal cord, energizes the inner cells, and activates the whole nervous system.

PAWANA MUKTA ASANA
(KNEE TO CHEST POSE)

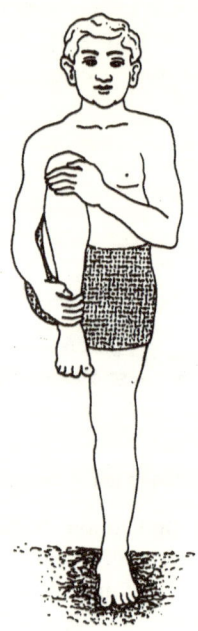

Figure 5.   Pawana Mukta Asana

Position of Readiness: Stand up. Keep both hands hanging down. Look straight ahead.

Steps of Actual Practice: (i) Lift one knee up towards the chest.

(ii) Put the same side hand on the ankle and the other hand on the knee as shown in Figure 5.

(iii) Bring the knee towards the chest without pulling on the ankle.

(iv) Stand firmly on the other leg, keeping it quite straight.

(v) Stay in that position for six to eight seconds, then release the knee and lower the leg.

(vi) Rest for six seconds and repeat the same process with the other leg.

Daily Practice: Six to eight times daily (three to four times with each knee alternately).

Note: Those who find it difficult to perform this *asana* while standing, may do it lying on the back. The method of practice is the same as in the standing position.

Benefits: It activates the pancreas and other abdominal organs mildly and effectively. It also relieves wind. For people suffering from wind trouble, acidity, and gas, it has an instant corrective effect. It loosens the hip joints and activates all the abdominal muscles and intestines. As a result of this internal activation, it cures constipation and corrects any malfunctioning of the stomach. Because of these internal effects, it helps to restore the functioning of the pancreas. It is an easy and harmless *asana;* anyone can do it.

BHUJANGA ASANA
(COBRA POSE)

Position of Readiness: Lie on the stomach. Let the head rest on either cheek. Bring the palms beneath the shoulders on both sides. The tips of the fingers should be at the edge of the

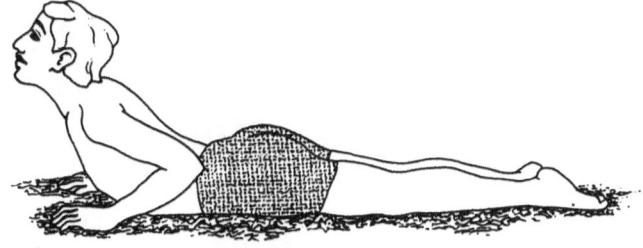

Figure 6. Bhujanga Asana

shoulders. The elbows should be folded upward close to the body. Keep the heels together and the toes flat on the floor. Breathe normally.

Steps of Actual Practice: (i) Straighten the head and tilt it slightly backward.

(ii) Inhaling slowly, raise your head and chest upwards so that, while your navel is on the floor, the portion above it is raised. In this position, both legs should be fully stretched and kept tightly together (Figure 6).

(iii) Then look up as far as you can and hold your breath for six to eight seconds.

(iv) After six to eight seconds, start exhaling and lowering the head towards the floor and let the head rest on either cheek.

(v) Now let the body relax and rest for six seconds.

(vi) After resting, repeat the process.

Daily Practice: Four times only.

Benefits: *Bhujanga asana* inwardly activates the entire abdominal area. Because of this activation, the pancreas, liver, and other organs of the digestive system are strengthened and normalized. It is regarded as one of the best *asanas* for eliminating constipation, indigestion, dysentery, wind troubles, stomachache, and other abdominal disorders. It makes the spine flexible and corrects spinal disorders and backache. It activates the chest, shoulders, neck, face, and head areas effectively and enhances facial beauty.

This *asana* has some specific benefits for women—various menstrual problems are corrected by it.

SHALABHA ASANA
(LOCUST POSE)

Position of Readiness: Lie on your stomach with either cheek on the floor. Stretch the hands on both sides of the body and keep them close to the thighs. Keep the thumb and index finger

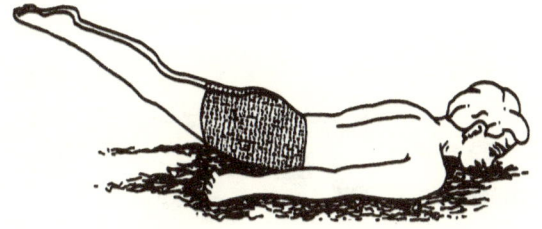

Figure 7.   Shalabha Asana

side of the palms down on the floor and make fists with both hands. Stretch both legs and let the toes be flat on the floor. Keep the heels and toes together. Make the whole body straight. Breathe normally.

Steps of Actual Practice: (i) Inhale slowly but deeply through both nostrils and hold the breath.

(ii) Lift the head slightly, straighten it, and then let the chin rest on the floor (use a folded towel underneath the chin).

(iii) Clench the fists and tense the arms and hands.

(iv) Now tighten both legs and lift them up together quickly as high as you easily can.

(v) Stay in that position for at least five to six seconds, keeping the legs tense (Figure 7).

(vi) Then slowly exhale while simultaneously lowering the legs towards the floor.

(vii) When the legs have touched the floor, turn the head and let it rest on either cheek; loosen the whole body.

(viii) Rest for five seconds and then repeat the *asana*.

Daily Practice: Only four times. (Do it after performing the *Bhujanga asana* for four times.)

Note: Those who feel it difficult to lift both legs together should lift only one leg at a time (Figure 8) for a few weeks. In this case, practice six rounds alternately, three times with each leg.

Benefits: This *asana* activates the kidneys, liver, pancreas, and

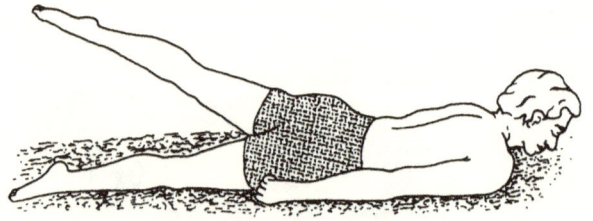

Figure 8. Shalabha Asana With One Leg at a Time

the whole abdominal area. Because of this internal activation, it removes constipation, wind troubles, indigestion, dysentery, diarrhea, acidity, and gastrointestinal disorders.

This *asana* also brings flexibility to the spine and invigorates the eyes, face, lungs, chest, neck, shoulders, and the whole upper area of the body. Since it is a harmless *asana*, it is recommended for every practitioner.

PASHCHIMOTTAN ASANA
(POSTERIOR STRETCH POSE)

Position of Readiness: Sit on the floor and stretch both legs in

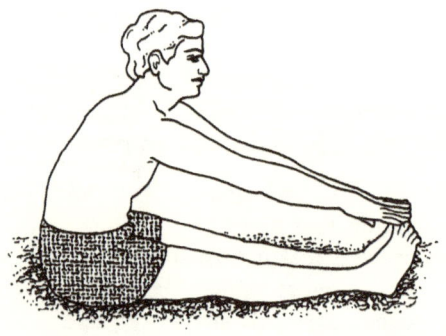

Figure 9. Readiness for Pashchimottan Asana

front. Keep the heels and toes together. Be seated firmly, with the spine, neck, and head straight. At this stage, the hands should be on the floor on both sides of the legs.

Steps of Actual Practice: (i) Stretch out both hands parallel to the stretched legs.

(ii) Touch the right toes with the fingers of the right hand and the left toes with those of the left hand (Figure 9). If you cannot touch the toes, go only as far as you can while keeping both legs stretched and the palms down. Do not bend or lift the knees.

(iii) Bow your head downward until it is between the two arms. Exhale all air out by the time the head is down.

(iv) Stretch the toes and tighten the legs and, while keeping the head between the arms, stretch both hands as far forward as possible. Without bending the legs at the knee, stay in that position for six to eight seconds (Figure 10).

(v) Now drop both palms on the legs and start inhaling and returning to the position of readiness. Draw the palms over the legs while returning to the seated position.

(vi) Rest for five seconds and repeat the process.

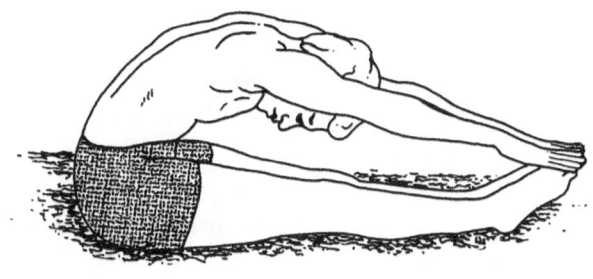

Figure 10. Pashchimottan Asana

Daily Practice: Four times daily. (Practice at least three times and at most five times a day.)

Note: Those who have had a back injury or spinal disorder with severe pain are advised to practice lightly and comfortably without forcing the body to bend excessively.

Benefits: This *asana* affects the whole spinal cord, the complete nervous system, and all the abdominal organs and glands. As a result, disorders of these parts are corrected. It has a curative effect for diabetics because it activates the pancreas and the endocrine glands. This activation regularizes the functioning of the pancreas so that it begins to secrete insulin normally.

This *asana* also corrects backache, cures spinal disorders, relieves stomach troubles, and normalizes the functioning of the nervous system.

It might not be possible for many people to do this *asana* accurately. They are advised to do only as much of it as they can comfortably. In due course, after practicing for a while, they will improve and will begin to do it properly. Since this is a very beneficial *asana*, it is recommended to every practitioner.

Remember: The method of doing an *asana* is more important than repeating it a number of times.

SHAVA ASANA
(RELAXATION POSE)

Position of Readiness: Lie on your back. Keep the whole body loose and straight. The palms can be either up or down on the floor. Do not use any pillow under your head. At this point, breathe normally. Keep the eyes closed and let the whole body fall on the floor in an unrestrained way. This is the position of readiness and remains the same during the actual practice (Figure 11).

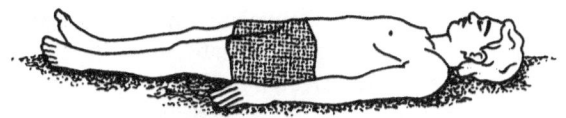

Figure 11. Shava Asana

Steps of Actual Practice: (i) Close your eyes and keep them closed for two seconds. Then open them for two seconds. Do this simple opening and closing of the eyes three to four times.

(ii) Open the eyes again and look upward for two seconds, then downward for two seconds, then straight. Now look towards the left for two seconds, then towards the right for two seconds, then straight ahead again, and then close the eyes. Repeat this eye exercise two to three times.

(iii) Now open your mouth wide without straining it. Turn the tongue so that its tip is folded back towards the throat and then close the mouth. Keep the mouth closed and tongue folded for ten seconds. Then open the mouth, bring the tongue back to its normal position, and then close the mouth. Repeat this process two to three times.

(iv) Keeping your eyes closed, bring your mental attention towards your toes. See (mentally) that the toes are relaxed. Then move slowly up towards the head mentally by checking the knees, thighs, waist, spinal cord, back, shoulders, neck, arms, palms, fingers, and the rest of the body to be sure that they are actually relaxed. Now, move the neck and head slightly to the right and left. Then let the head rest in a comfortable position. Now the entire body is physically relaxed.

(v) Relax the mind by the following process:

Select a place of natural beauty which you have visited and liked, such as a park, a garden, a beach, or a riverside, and feel as if you are mentally present there. Attach your mind to that place. Imagine that you are lying there and breathing the air of the same environment. Now, while keeping the mind in that environment, exhale and inhale slowly but deeply. During the breathing, the stomach should rise while inhaling and lower while exhaling. One exhalation and inhalation make one round. Do not rush in this deep breathing. Do it about ten to twelve times. When the deep breathing is over, feel as if you are going to sleep and relax completely. Stay in that position for five to ten minutes. Then open your eyes, stretch your body, and slowly be seated. You have completed the *Shava asana*.

Daily Practice: Do *Shava asana* at the end of all *asanas*, *pranayamas*, and other *kriyas* for ten to fifteen minutes daily. In certain cases like hypertension and heart trouble, *Shava asana* should be performed singly for longer periods without practicing any other *asanas* or *kriyas*.

Benefits: *Shava asana* has a very good effect upon a patient as well as upon any yoga practitioner. One immediate effect is that it relaxes all the muscles, nerves, the body's organs, and the mind. When the muscles, nerves, and organs are fully relaxed, they regain their strength and normal health is restored.

For people suffering from insomnia; high and low blood pressure; gastric, lung, and heart troubles; and mental illness, this *asana* is remarkable for providing immediate relief. Those who suffer from fatigue and a lack of vitality will find that this *asana* gives energy and strength. Because of these good effects, every practitioner of yoga is advised to perform it daily.

CHAPTER 3

Diabetes

DIABETES is a very old disease and millions all over the world suffer from it. Although the symptoms and nature of diabetes vary, its common feature is that there is excessive sugar in the blood and this sugar is evident in the urine. This excessive accumulation of sugar in the blood is caused by the malfunctioning of the pancreas.

When the pancreas—a gland situated in the upper side of the abdomen—does not produce enough insulin, the body fails to utilize sugar and create energy from it. When this sugar is not properly used, the body's chemistry is disturbed and the individual develops various physical ailments and disorders. Consequently, there is frequent urination, excessive thirst, fatigue, loss of weight, blurred vision, general weakness, and skin disorders. Further, with chronicity, hypertension (high blood pressure) and kidney disorders also develop. The usual method of treating the diabetic is to inject insulin to compensate for what cannot be produced by the pancreas.

The main problem with medicinal treatment is that the

patient must keep taking injections and other medicines indefinitely and the disease is still not eliminated.

Yoga Treatment: The yoga system of treatment consists of proper diet and regular yoga practice. Initially, the patient can start yoga practice without stopping the medicine or injections if he is under medical treatment. After practicing yoga for about three weeks, the person should *gradually* reduce and finally stop taking the medicines.

While treating diabetic patients at the Indian Institute of Yoga, we have found that it takes from two to three months to cure this disease.[1]

The yogic treatment restores the normal functioning of the pancreas and other endocrinal glands. When these glands begin to function properly, the body chemistry becomes normal, the individual is fully cured of the diabetic disorders, and his health is restored to normal.

Proper Diet: It is important for persons suffering from diabetes to avoid fried, fatty, spicy, starchy, and sugar-containing food. For four months from the date of starting yoga practices, diabetic patients *should not eat* rice, potatoes, bananas, grapes, oranges, mangoes, and other fruits in which the percentage of sugar is high. Vegetarians can take wheat bread, legumes, green vegetables, salad, leafy vegetables, germinated beans, and cheese. They can eat an apple a day. Non-vegetarians may add small quantities of fish, liver, and egg to their diets, but should avoid meat or chicken for a few months.

Diabetics are generally overweight. If they follow the principles and ways of eating as mentioned in Chapter 1 and keep practicing yoga, this extra weight will be automatically reduced. The point to remember is that they must take their

---

[1]We have found that diabetes among people over forty years of age is cured sooner than among people below forty. Juvenile diabetes (occurring in those under twenty years of age) may take about a year or more for complete cure.

evening meals at least two hours before going to bed and must always eat less than eighty-five percent of their capacity. A diet chart for diabetics is given below:

Breakfast (7 to 9 A.M.)

(i)	Apple or peach	— one or half
	or	
	Tomato or vegetable juice	— ½ glass
(ii)	Sprouted chick-peas	— one handful
(iii)	Whole wheat bread	— one or two slices
	or	
	Wheat germ or wheat cereal (with skim milk)	— one cup
(iv)	Egg	— one boiled, if desired
(v)	Herb tea or decaffeinated coffee	— one cup, if necessary, without sugar or honey

Lunch and Dinner (12 noon to 2 P.M. and 6 to 8 P.M.)

(i)	Salad (a mixture of cucumber, tomato, lettuce, radish, watercress, celery, and sprouts) with unsweetened salad dressing or with a little salt, pepper, and lemon juice	— as desired
(ii)	Vegetable, tomato, or bean soup	— medium soup bowl
(iii)	Whole wheat bread	— as desired
(iv)	Vegetables (any kind)	— as desired
(v)	Leafy vegetables (any kind)	— as desired
(vi)	Beans (of any kind) or green peas	— as desired
(vii)	Fish or liver (for non-vegetarians)	— if desired
(viii)	Low-fat yogurt or buttermilk	— if desired

Afternoon Refreshments (3 to 4 P.M.)

(i) Apple, papaya, or peach	— one or half
(ii) Crackers	— one or two
(iii) Raw nuts (a mixture of cashews, pecans, pistachios, walnuts, and almonds—not fried or roasted)	— one handful
(iv) Herb tea or decaffeinated coffee	— one cup, if desired, without sugar or honey

Relevant Asanas: Since the main problem here is to restore the normal functioning of the pancreas and some other glands, the first consideration is to select those *asanas* which can help to revive the normal functioning of the endocrinal system. Secondly, we should choose such *asanas* which can easily be practiced by all. Accordingly, the *asanas* we recommend are: *Surya Namaskar asana, Uttanapada asana, Bhujanga asana, Shalabha asana, Pashchimottan asana, Ardha Vakra asana, Matsyendra asana, Supta Vajra asana, Dhanur asana,* and *Shava asana.* A regular practice of even six to seven of these *asanas* would be enough to cure diabetes.

SURYA NAMASKAR ASANA
(BOWING BEFORE THE SUN POSE)

Position of Readiness: Stand up with the legs about two feet apart. Let the hands hang loosely at your sides. Keep the head straight. Look directly in front and breathe normally.

Steps of Actual Practice: (i) Inhale slowly and raise both arms from the sides to above the head. Time it so that, by the time your hands are above your head, you also complete inhaling. When the hands are up, the palms should be turned forward and the arms should be parallel.

(ii) Start exhaling and bending the upper area of the body

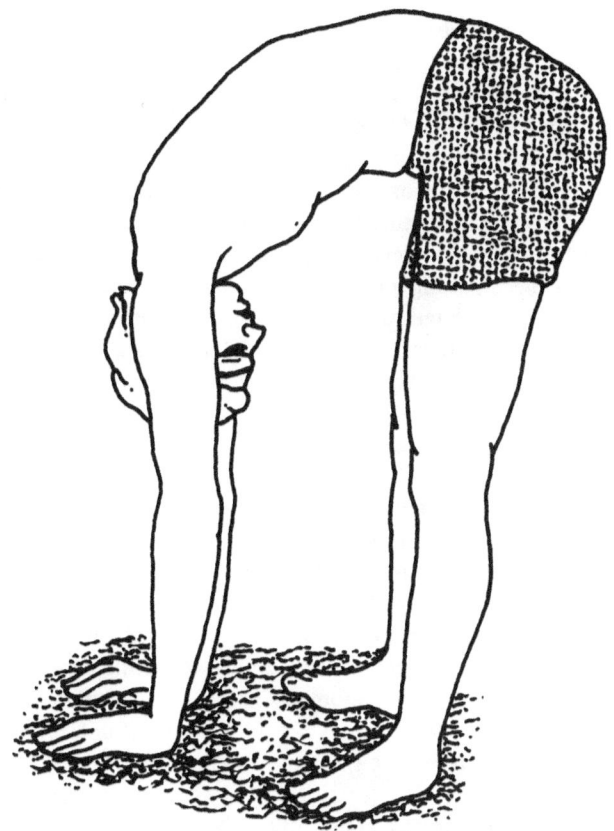

Figure 12.   Surya Namaskar Asana

towards the floor. While bending forward, stretch the arms and keep both hands parallel to each other and move them towards the floor in front of you. By the time both hands reach, or almost reach, the floor, you should have finished exhaling.

(iii) Now hold the breath and stay in this position for about six to eight seconds. While holding your breath, it is important that you keep the upper part of the body (above the waist) quite loose, and the lower part (i.e., below the waist) tense. Bend your head so that the top of it is towards the ground. Your head should be between the arms. Hands should hang loosely as far down as they can easily go. If you can, put the palms on the floor or just touch the floor. It is important that you not strain yourself or force your body excessively while bending. Do only as much as you can comfortably (Figure 12).

(iv) Place both hands on the legs and inhale and come up to the standing position, letting the palms pass over and touch the legs upwardly. Inhale slowly so that by the time you have returned to the standing position you have finished inhaling. Now you have completed one round of *Surya Namaskar asana*.

(v) Rest for five to six seconds and then repeat the same process. Stay in the position of readiness while resting.

Daily Practice: Four times only.

Benefits: This *asana* activates almost all the glands of the endocrine system in a mild way. Because of this activation, the pancreas, adrenal, thyroid, pituitary, and some other glands begin to secrete their respective hormones normally. Since the main trouble with diabetics results from a malfunctioning pancreas, this *asana* corrects its defects by activating it.

It has good effects on the stomach, spine, lungs, and chest. Various disorders in these areas are corrected by this *asana*. Because there is a reverse circulation of the blood during this *asana*, it invigorates the facial tissues, the central nervous system, and all the organs of the upper body. It is easy to do and is therefore recommended to all practitioners of yoga.

After performing the *Surya Namaskar asana*, the following *asanas* should be gradually added to the daily practice:

Uttanapada asana:	Figures 3 and 4
Bhujanga asana:	Figure 6
Shalabha asana:	Figures 7 and 8
Pashchimottan asana:	Figures 9 and 10

All four *asanas* are fully described in Chapter 2. Diabetic patients are advised to practice these *asanas* exactly as described.

ARDHA VAKRA ASANA
(TWIST POSE)

Position of Readiness: Sit on the floor. Stretch both legs in front, parallel to each other. Put both palms on the floor. Breathe normally. Keep the back straight while sitting.

Steps of Actual Practice: (i) Let one leg remain stretched on the floor; bend the other leg at the knee and pull it slightly backward.

(ii) Put the heel of the folded leg at the central point between the knee and the ankle of the stretched leg. Then drop the heel on the outer side of the leg. Keep the heel quite close to the stretched leg. The knee of your bent leg should be upward.

(iii) Lift the hand which is on the side of the stretched leg; bring it up and parallel to the stretched leg. Grasp the stretched leg near the heel of the bent leg. Now you have made a lock with the arm and the knee. If you cannot hold the stretched leg, just touch it or keep the fingers near its center.

(iv) Lift the other hand and place its palm on the waist, keeping the thumb and the index finger side upward. Now your elbow is folded and making a 90-degree angle with the stretched leg. At this stage, see that your head, neck, and back are straight up.

(v) Start exhaling slowly and at the same time begin twisting and turning the waist, chest, neck, and head in the direction of the bent elbow. Twist and turn as much as you can comfortably. In this turn, your folded elbow travels 90 degrees, but the head and the upper area of the body travel 180 degrees. For example, if you were sitting facing east and you have to turn right, then your face will first turn south and then west while your stretched leg will remain facing east.

(vi) After turning as much as you can, hold the breath and stay in that position for six to eight seconds. At this stage, your spine should be straight and you should be projecting the vision at a maximum distance (Figure 13).

(vii) Then start inhaling slowly and return to the position of readiness.

(viii) Now break the lock, stretch out the legs, relax the body, put the palms on the floor, and rest for six seconds.

(ix) After resting, repeat the *asana* with the other leg, following the same method.

Daily Practice: Four to six rounds alternately. Never do it more than six times (three times with each side).

Benefits: The main effect of this *asana* is on the waist and

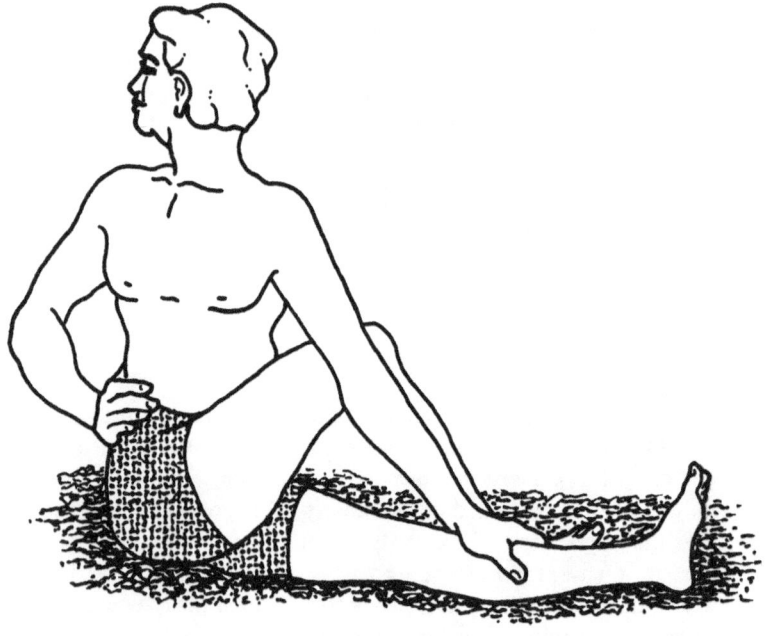

Figure 13. Ardha Vakra Asana

abdominal areas. It activates all the organs and glands of these parts of the body. This *asana* has a very good effect on the pancreas, adrenal glands, ovaries in women, and the testicles in men.

It has several other benefits: It corrects constipation, stomach troubles, piles, backache, stiffness in the neck, and spinal disorders. It is easy to do and is therefore recommended to every yoga practitioner.

MATSYENDRA ASANA
(FULL TWIST POSE)

Matsyendra asana is a little difficult. It may not be possible for everyone to do it perfectly at first. But, since it is an important *asana*, practitioners are advised to do only as much of it as they can quite comfortably. Those who can practice *Matsyendra asana* perfectly well should not practice *Ardha Vakra asana* because both have a similar effect. Since *Ardha Vakra asana* is easier to do, practitioners should begin with it first.

Position of Readiness: Be seated on the floor and stretch both legs in front. Keep the legs parallel. Put the palms on the floor on both sides of the body. Straighten the body. Look in front and breathe normally.

Steps of Actual Practice: (i) Bend the right leg at the knee by pulling it backward. Now the right thigh is standing upward and the right buttock has been raised. At this stage, keep the right leg where it is.

(ii) Bend the left leg at the knee without lifting it. The thigh and knee of the left leg should remain on the floor and the foot should be brought below the right buttock. The left foot may be gently pulled by hand to bring it underneath the buttock.

(iii) Now lift the right foot slightly and bring it on the outer side of the folded (bent) left knee. Keep the right foot quite close to the bent left knee. Now your right knee is standing upward and the left knee is on the floor.

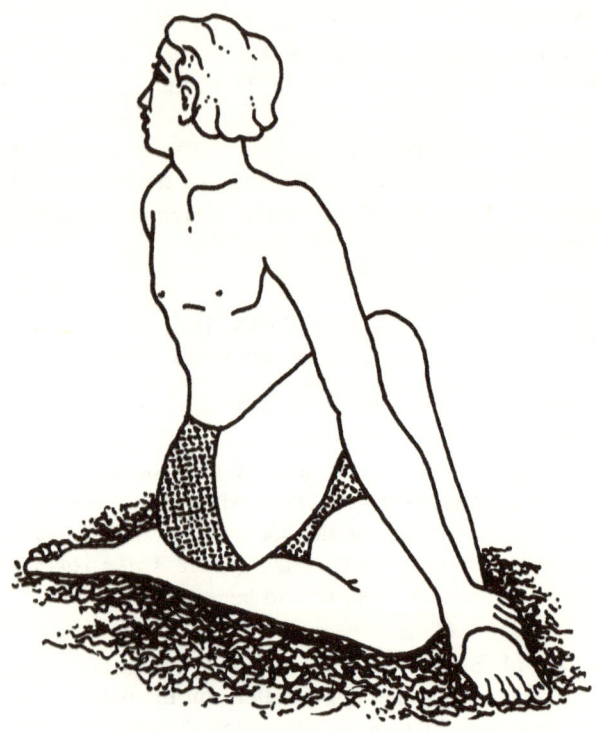

Figure 14.   Matsyendra Asana

(iv) Then you have to make a lock with the opposite arm and the standing knee. Since your right knee is standing, you have to make the lock with the left arm. Therefore, stretch out the left arm and bring it on the outer side of the right knee. Now your arm is locked against the standing knee firmly. Grab the right foot with the left hand to stabilize the locked part of the body.

(v) Bring the entire right arm and hand on the back loosely. Try to touch the front part of the waist with the fingers of the hand on the back. You are now ready to make the turn. At this stage, be sure that your spine, neck, and head are in a straight upward position.

(vi) Begin exhaling slowly and turning the head, chest, and waist areas towards the right side. Twist the body as much as you can. Be sure that all the air has been expelled by the time you have made the full twist. Look back as far as you can. Keep the back straight upward. You should be in the same position as shown in Figure 14.

(vii) Stay in that position for six to eight seconds. The holding time may be for only four to six seconds in the beginning stage of practice.

(viii) Then start inhaling slowly and gradually return to the position from which you started the twist. You have completed one round of *Matsyendra asana*.

(ix) Now unlock the arm and the knee, and be seated in the position of readiness and rest for six to eight seconds. During the rest, inhale and exhale deeply two times.

(x) After the rest, prepare to turn to the left side in another round. Now your left knee will be upward and your right arm will be locked. You must do it alternately.

Daily Practice: Four to six rounds alternately (three times with each side).

Benefits: This *asana* greatly affects the pancreas and other glands such as the adrenal, thyroid, and sex glands. The muscles and organs of the abdominal area are fully activated by this *asana*. Because of this activation, the condition and functioning of the pancreas are energized and strengthened. This is the reason why people suffering from diabetes are advised to practice this *asana* daily, even if they cannot do it quite properly.

This *asana* has several other benefits for any yoga practitioner. It corrects disorders of the kidneys, spleen, liver, stomach, intestines, bladder, and the pelvis because of the internal activation by this *asana*.

It also has a good effect on the lungs because blood circulation is improved by this *asana*. People with shortness of breath are advised to begin this *asana* in a mild way and gradually develop it to perfection.

This *asana* has some specific benefits in cases of spinal disorders. It removes rigidity of the spine and restores its flexibility. Since it twists the whole spinal cord from the back of the neck to the coccyx mildly and effectively, disorders of the whole spine are corrected.

Since this is a very beneficial *asana* for the diabetic patient, as well as for others, practitioners are advised to do it.

SUPTA VAJRA ASANA
(PELVIC POSE)

Position of Readiness: Sit on the floor with your legs folded under you (Figure 15). Put the palms on the floor on both sides of the body and straighten your spine. Now look in front and breathe normally.

Note: This *asana* is a little difficult. Those whose bodies are not very flexible are advised to practice this *asana* gradually without trying to do the complete *asana* all at once. By doing it in stages, it can be done without any strain.

Steps of Actual Practice: (i) Kneel on the floor, keeping the body weight on both knees. Put the palms on the floor on both sides of the bent knees to support some of the body's weight. Keep the knees about four inches apart from each other. Let the ankles and toes of both legs fall on the floor so that the toes are brought close together but the heels are spread out. This will make a broad "V" curve with the toes, soles, and heels.

(ii) Now gradually and cautiously start lowering the hips and let them rest on the curve of the soles. Control the body weight by keeping both hands on the floor while lowering the hips. If you do not feel strained, put the weight of the whole body on the curve of the feet as shown in Figure 15. If there is difficulty in sitting in this position, further stages should not be tried until the body is prepared for it. Those who can sit comfortably on the toes and soles should proceed to the third stage.

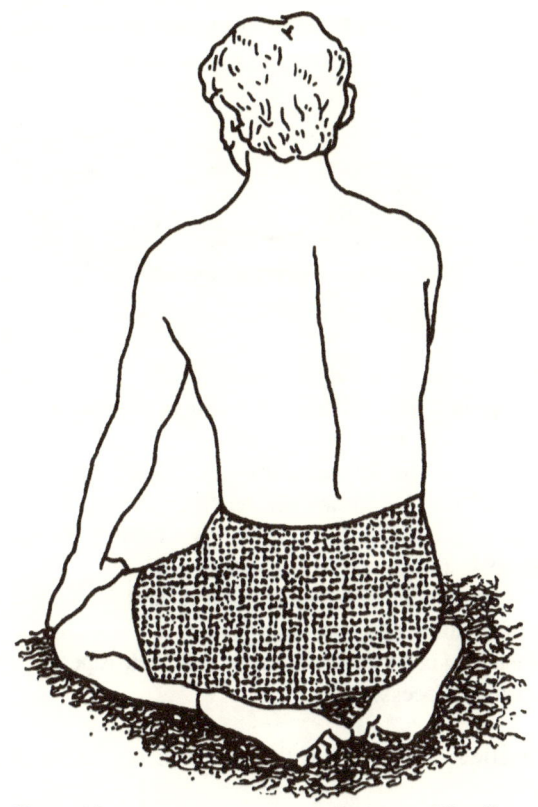

Figure 15.   Supta Vajra Asana (Position of Readiness)

(iii) Place the right hand on the floor behind the hip. Then move the left hand also behind the hip and bend a little backward.

(iv) Now put the right elbow on the floor by bending backward. Then put the left elbow on the floor. While moving the elbows towards the hips, gradually let the head touch the floor. When the head has reached the floor, gradually put the shoulders and then the whole back of your body on the floor. Do not rush. Go slow in this process.

(v) Now stretch both the arms and hands on both sides of the body. Keep the palms on the floor and close to the body, as shown in Figure 16.

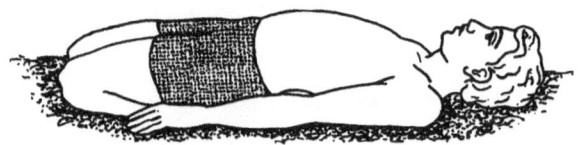

Figure 16. Supta Vajra Asana

(vi) Then do a few deep breathings by just inhaling and exhaling through both nostrils. Remain in this position for six to eight seconds or less.

(vii) Return by the following method: Grasp the ankles with the hands and put the elbows on the floor. Now pull the ankles and, by putting the weight of the body on the elbows, lift the head and back and return to the sitting position.

(viii) Then unwind the bended knees and be seated in the position of readiness to rest.

(ix) Rest for six to eight seconds and then repeat the *asana* with the same process.

Daily Practice: Three to four times. Never do it more than five times.

Benefits: This *asana* has some special benefits for people suffering from diabetes. Since this *asana* activates all the cells of the pancreas and increases its blood supply, the pancreas begins to function normally. This *asana* has several other benefits: It corrects disorders of the stomach, intestines, liver, kidneys, spleen, and all the organs of the abdominal area by activating and energizing them.

It has medicinal value for people suffering from indigestion, wind trouble, constipation, and piles. Disorders of the spine and joints are effectively corrected by this *asana*. It also has a good effect on the sex glands and enhances sexual potency.

DHANUR ASANA
(BOW POSE)

Position of Readiness: Lie on your stomach. Keep your arms stretched on both sides. Rest your head on either cheek on the floor. Bring the legs and heels together. Breathe normally. Bend both legs at the knees and bring the heels close to your hips. Then grasp the right ankle with the right hand and the left ankle with the left hand. If you find it difficult to reach the ankles, you may hold the toes. Now, holding either the ankles or the toes firmly, bring the knees and the ankles close together. Keep the cheek on the floor.

Steps of Actual Practice: (i) Inhale slowly but deeply and hold the breath.

(ii) When the inhaling is over, lift the head up and straighten it.

(iii) Without waiting any longer, give a backward pull with both legs. Do not rush in giving the backward pull; do it slowly but constantly and smoothly. Let the legs go backward as much as they can. This will raise your chest, neck, and head upward.

(iv) Look upwards, keeping the knees close to one another and on the floor. Do not lift the knees from the floor. Keep the

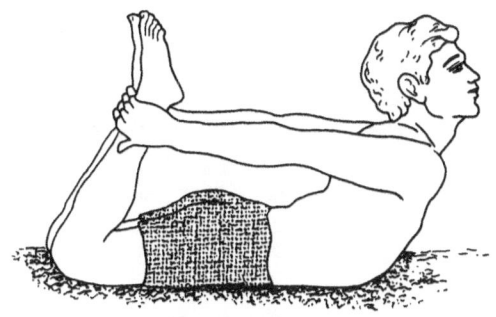

Figure 17. Dhanur Asana

ankles together, if possible. Remain in this position for six to eight seconds while holding the breath. You should be in the position shown in Figure 17.

(v) Start exhaling and simultaneously lowering the head and chest towards the floor.

(vi) Let your head rest on the floor, on either cheek. Release the ankles and let them fall back slowly on the floor. Bring the hands to the floor and relax.

(vii) After resting for six to eight seconds, repeat the *asana* as before.

Daily Practice: Three to four times only. Those who might find it difficult to do the complete *asana* by holding both the ankles should practice with only one ankle at a time for a few days. In this case, the whole process of inhaling, rising, holding, and returning is the same as done with both ankles. The only difference is that one leg remains stretched on the floor while the other is bent, held, and pulled. It is very easy to do with one ankle at a time.

Benefits: *Dhanur asana* activates all the glands of the endocrinal system. The pancreas becomes fully energized because of the internal as well as external impact of this *asana* on it. Thus, there is an all-round conditioning of the pancreas. As a result, its normal health is restored and it begins to release insulin properly.

The *asana* has a good effect on the adrenal, thyroid, parathyroid, pituitary, and sex glands. Because the cells of all these glands are activated, the secretion of their respective hormones becomes normal.

This *asana* corrects disorders of the joints, spinal cord, lungs, chest, and abdomen. It removes various types of stomach troubles, develops digestive power, and eliminates extra weight and fat.

The *asana* has some specific benefits for women: It corrects menstrual disorders and other troubles related to the reproductive organs.

CHAPTER 4

Asthma

THE most common symptom of asthma is breathlessness, which is caused by the disorder and bronchial spasms in the respiratory system. The asthmatic strains just to get a breath. In severe cases, the life of the patient becomes miserable and the condition almost makes him an invalid.

Asthma is mainly a disorder of the bronchioles which are constricted, thus disturbing the normal ratio of inhalation and expiration. Because the blood vessels of the bronchial lining are congested, expiration becomes prolonged and difficult.

This is a widely prevalent disease, affecting the young, old, and even children. The most disheartening aspect of asthma is that it does not get completely cured through medicines.

In treating patients of asthma at the Indian Institute of Yoga at Patna, we have had very satisfactory results. The patients who followed our instructions well and practiced yoga regularly were cured. The health of both male and female patients became normal with a few months of their yoga practice and there was no recurrence of it among the cured ones.

The yoga system of treatment for this disease requires three things: (i) practicing *pranayama* and selected *asanas* regularly, (ii) eating a proper diet, and (iii) observing certain principles and suggestions.

Pranayama and Asanas: Because asthma is primarily a disease of the lungs and the respiratory system, the *pranayama* and *asanas* must be so selected that their practice will restore normal health to the lungs and the entire respiratory system. With this aim in mind, I recommend the following *pranayama* and *asanas:*

Ujjayee Pranayama, Ekpada Utthan asana, Tara asana, Yoga Mudra, Ushtra asana, Simha asana, Sarvanga asana, Matsya asana, Padma asana, and Shava asana.

Proper Diet: Asthmatics should eat a daily balanced diet which includes salad, fresh fruits, green vegetables, germinated chick-peas, wheat bread, and leafy vegetables. They should eat four times a day: breakfast, lunch, afternoon refreshment, and dinner.

Breakfast should consist of some fruit juice, fresh fruits, a handful of germinated chick-peas, wheat bread, and green vegetables.

Lunch and dinner should begin with about a cup of salad (slices of cucumber, lettuce, tomato, carrot, beets, and any other vegetable which can be eaten raw). The salad should be mixed with salt, pepper, and lemon juice or with salad dressing. After eating salad, patients should eat soup (if possible), wheat bread, any kind of leafy vegetable, and some fresh green vegetables. Non-vegetarians can eat fish and liver if they like. Meat of any other type should be avoided for three months.

In the afternoon, some light refreshment should be taken, such as fresh fruits, cheese, or crackers.

Principles and Suggestions: It is very important that asthmatics follow the following principles and suggestions in their diet and daily life.

They must eat dinner at least two hours before going to bed at night. They should never eat more than eighty-five percent of their stomach's capacity at any time. They should eat slowly and chew the food properly, drink water after half an hour of finishing their meals, take ten to twelve glasses of water in a day, and avoid hot spices, red pepper, and pickles. Their intake of tea or coffee should not be more than two cups in a day. They should not take tea in the morning, and they should not drink water upon arising and before going to the toilet.

Asthmatics should avoid diets and such ways of living to which they are allergic. They should cut down on or give up cigarettes and the use of tobacco in any form. If it is difficult to give up smoking, they should not smoke on an empty stomach. They should sleep six to eight hours daily and should try to be relaxed rather than tense. Those conditions which cause nervousness and tension should be corrected and eliminated. Asthmatics are strongly advised to bathe daily with either cold or hot water, to rub the whole body with a rough towel, and to use bathing soap. They should avoid massaging the body daily with any oil. They should maintain neatness and cleanliness as much as possible. With these guidelines, they should practice the following *pranayama* and *asanas*.

UJJAYEE PRANAYAMA
(IN LYING POSITION)

Pranayama is mainly a *kriya* (exercise) with air. As we know, air possesses several unique qualities. It contains "life force" (*Prana shakti*). It also has an absorbing, activating, and massaging capacity. Because of these qualities, air is regarded as a great purifier as well as a giver of life to the inner organs of the body. The body makes full use of these qualities during *pranayama*.[1]

---

[1]For a comprehensive understanding of the scientific values of *pranayama*, see Dr. Phulgenda Sinha, *Yoga: Meaning, Values and Practice* (Patna: Indian Institute of Yoga, 1970), pp 77-85; Swami Kuvalayananda, *Pranayama* (Bombay: Popular Prakashan, 1972).

Ujjayee Pranayama can be practiced in two positions: standing and lying. There is full impact of it in the first position and a little less in the second. But the first is a little strenuous and the second is easier. Therefore, practitioners are advised to practice *Ujjayee* lying down for one month and then may switch to the standing position (as described next), if preferred.

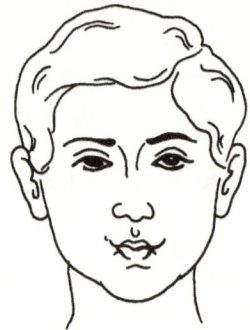

Figure 18.   Exhalation in Ujjayee Pranayama

Position of Readiness: Lie on your back on the floor. Make the body straight. Put the palms on the floor and close to the body. Bring the heels together and keep the legs loose. Look straight upward and breathe normally.

Steps of Actual Practice: There are four steps in *Ujjayee*:
    (i) Exhaling the air through the mouth;
    (ii) Inhaling through both nostrils;
    (iii) Retaining the air; and
    (iv) Exhaling the air again through the mouth.

These steps must be performed in the sequence described below:

(i) Exhale all the air of the body through the mouth as continuously and rapidly as you would when whistling. Expel the air through the lips without twisting any facial tissues (Figure 18).

During this stage, the body should remain loose. The abdomen should be contracted during exhalation. When all the air has been exhaled, begin the second stage immediately.

(ii) Inhale air slowly through both nostrils. Do not rush. Fill the body by as much air as can be inhaled comfortably. Do not try to inhale excessively. Keep the body loose at this stage. The inhalation will make the abdominal area expand.

(iii) When inhalation is completed, retain the air and do the following: Bring the toes of both legs together and stretch them forward. Tighten the legs. Pull the stomach gradually inwards. Keep the arms stretched. There should be a mild tightening of the muscles of the whole body. Remain in this position (as shown in Figure 19) for three to four seconds only during the

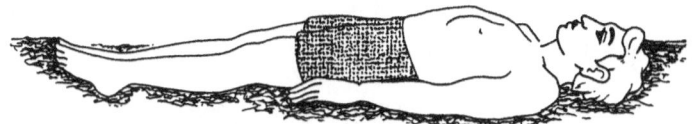

Figure 19. Retention in Ujjayee in Lying Position

first week. Gradually increase the retention time to six or eight seconds during the second or third week. The principle is to retain only as long as you can do it comfortably.

(iv) After retaining for the desired seconds, exhale through the mouth in the same way as you did during the first step. The air should be released steadily and continuously but in a controlled way. Do not rush. While exhaling, start loosening the body muscles from the top downwards; that is, first loosen the chest, then the stomach, then the thighs, legs, and the arms. Relax the whole body as you fully exhale. You have made one round of *Ujjayee Pranayama*. Now rest for five to six seconds.

While resting, inhale and exhale normally through the nostrils. When the rest is over, repeat the same process as in the first round.

Daily Practice: On the first day of practice, perform it only three times. Increase to four times on the second day and then go to five times on the third day. Do not do it more than five times at a stretch. That is the maximum at one time. Those who wish to practice it twice a day should let eight hours elapse between the first and the second practice. Morning and evening are best suitable for twice-a-day practice.

Caution: *Pranayama* must be done on an empty stomach. The best time to do it is in the morning, after washing up. The second good time is in the evening. Those who would like to do it in the evening must give a gap of three to four hours after eating. This *pranayama* must be done where fresh air is available and when the body temperature is normal.

Benefits: Though a full description of its benefits is presented in the following pages, let me mention here that the practice of *Ujjayee Pranayama* in the lying position has all the same benefits as when done standing. It is important to note that it is safe and easy to do in the lying position. People with high and low blood pressure, those who take drugs habitually, and those with heart trouble are specially advised to practice it in this position until they feel quite normal.

UJJAYEE PRANAYAMA
(IN STANDING POSITION)

The method of practicing *Ujjayee Pranayama* lying down has been described earlier. Now the process of practicing it in the standing position is presented. But let me first caution you.

Caution: *Ujjayee Pranayama* in the standing position must be practiced *exactly* as described. Any laxity in following the instructions can cause injury and harm. Unless *Ujjavee*

Pranayama in the standing position is done properly, the practitioner might fall and injure himself. Therefore, it is strongly advised to obey the following guidelines while practicing *Ujjayee Pranayama* standing.

(i) Practice Ujjayee Pranayama first in the lying position for about a month, then try the standing position. There is no danger of injury and harm in the lying position.

(ii) *Ujjayee Pranayama* in the standing position must be practiced in fresh air, when the body is not tired, when the body temperature is normal, and when the practitioner is not in a hurry.

(iii) Every step must be done gradually and rhythmically.

Position of Readiness: Stand, join your heels, and spread your toes at a forty-five degree angle. Let the hands hang loosely on both sides. Look straight ahead at eye level. Stand firmly but without tightening the body. Be relaxed.

Steps of Actual Practice: There are four steps in the standing position of *Ujjayee Pranayama:* (i) exhaling air through the mouth; (ii) inhaling air through both nostrils; (iii) retaining the air; and (iv) exhaling the air again through the mouth. These four steps must be done in the sequence described below:

(i) Exhale all air through the mouth in a rapid and continuous way. The air is blown out through and between the lips (see Figure 18). The speed of the exhaled air during this step is the same as it is when you whistle. During this stage, keep the whole body loose. When you start exhaling, gradually pull in the stomach muscles (contract the stomach). When all the air has been expelled, begin the second stage without waiting.

(ii) Inhale slowly and continuously through both nostrils. Do not rush to finish inhaling quickly. Inhale without straining or twisting the facial muscles. Inhale only as much air as you can take quite comfortably. During inhalation, the body should remain loose. As the air is filled inside, the abdominal muscles should expand. In other words, let the abdominal area come forward as it would when you blow into a balloon.

(iii) When the inhaling is over, retain (hold) the air inside. For retaining, it is important that you start tightening the whole body gradually from the legs upwards to the chest. *Do not rush to retain all at once.*

Do the following process to properly condition your body during retention:

First tighten the muscles of the legs and then the thighs. Now gradually pull the stomach in only as much as you can comfortably. Raise the chest slightly forward. Bring the palms on the sides of the thighs and tighten the hands and arms. Look in front on the level of your eyes. Do not raise the shoulders. Slightly tighten the whole body; do not tighten excessively. Retain the air inside for only as long as you feel quite comfortable. Do not strain yourself too hard to hold the air (see

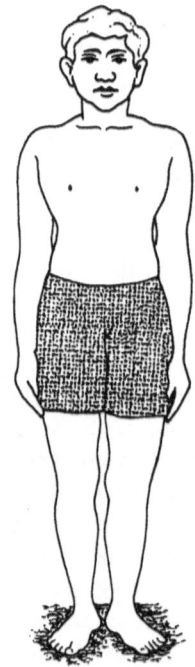

Figure 20.   Retention in Ujjayee in Standing Position

Figure 20). At the beginning stage of practice, hold your breath for two to three seconds only and gradually increase the holding time to six or eight seconds. Holding the breath for a very long time is not needed in *Ujjayee Pranayama*.

(iv) After retaining the air for the specified time, exhale through the mouth in a controlled but rapid manner. While exhaling, gradually start loosening the body from the chest downwards to the legs. Do not loosen the body quickly. First loosen the chest, then the abdominal muscles, then the thighs, legs, and hands. By the time you have completely exhaled, the body should also become loose. While exhaling, do not bend the head or chest either backward or forward. Keep standing straight. With this, one round of *Ujjayee* is completed. Now rest for six to eight seconds and inhale and exhale normally twice through the nostrils while keeping the mouth closed. When the rest is over, repeat the same process for further rounds.

Daily Practice: Begin with only three on the first day. Make four rounds on the second day and go to five rounds on the third. Five rounds are the maximum. Do not ever practice more than five rounds in a single session.

Benefits: The most remarkable benefit of *Ujjayee* is that it does the internal purification, activation, and energizing, together with external control and conditioning, all at the same time. For asthmatics, *Ujjayee* is most effective for correcting and strengthening the lungs and the bronchiole linings. To convey its benefits properly, let me explain what *Ujjayee* does to the internal organs of the body.

We know that air has an absorbing capacity. It can absorb certain things such as moisture, fragrance, and odors. Air also has the force and power to carry things such as dust particles and even heavier objects. We also know that, if we put air in a balloon and apply external pressure, the air would move and would try to penetrate even the minutest available space.

With this understanding about the nature of air, it can very easily be comprehended that, when the air is kept in the body for a longer time, it absorbs the impurities of the system and when it is expelled with a force it carries those inner impurities out. Further, when external pressure is applied, it maximizes the inner penetration of the air and enables it to rub, activate, and internally massage the body's cells and organs. This inner massage is a unique benefit of *Ujjayee* and hence is recommended highly for any adult practitioner of yoga.

EKPADA UTTHAN ASANA
(ONE LEG LIFT POSE)

In the preceding pages, the methods of practicing *Ujjayee Pranayama* have been fully explained. Asthmatics have been advised to practice five rounds of it daily in either a lying or standing position. After doing *Ujjayee*, they should practice the selected *asanas* as presented in this chapter. The first *asana* of this series is the *Ekpada Utthan asana*.

Position of Readiness: Lie down with your back on the floor. Keep the body straight. Bring the heels together. Keep the palms on the floor, close to the body. Let the body remain loose. Look straight upward and breathe normally.

Steps of Actual Practice: (i) Stretch out the toes of any one leg and tighten the leg muscles. Keep the other leg loose.

(ii) When the leg has been tightened, start inhaling and raising the leg upward. Inhale and raise the leg slowly, so that it should take about eight seconds to bring it upward to a perpendicular position. While lifting the leg, do not twist or turn the other parts of the body. Let the whole body remain on the floor. Lift the leg only as high as it can go comfortably. Do not strain excessively to push the leg up.

(iii) When the leg has been brought up to a maximum height, hold the breath and keep the leg firmly in the standing position. Retain the breath for six seconds only. During this stage of retention, be sure that your body is straight, the lifted

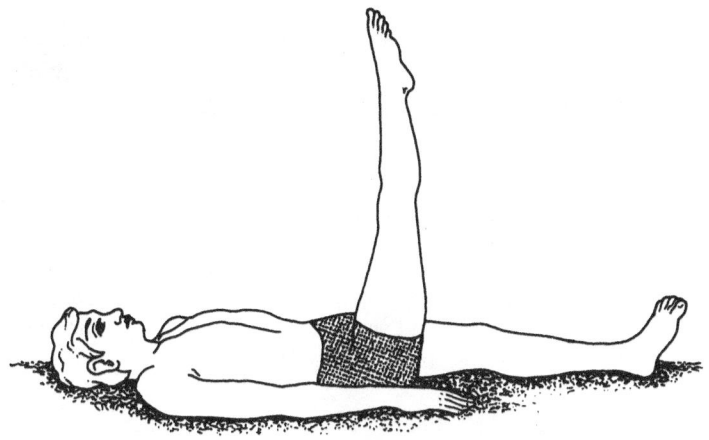

Figure 21. Ekpada Utthan Asana

leg is quite tight, palms are down on the floor, and you are looking upwards as shown in Figure 21.

(iv) After holding the breath for six seconds, start exhaling and lowering the leg towards the floor. It should take about eight seconds to complete exhalation. The leg should remain stiff and tight while it is brought down. When the leg reaches the floor, one round of *Ekpada Utthan asana* has been completed.

(v) Now rest for six to eight seconds. Then repeat the same process with the other leg.

Daily Practice: Begin with four rounds. Do it alternately. Gradually increase to six rounds.

Benefits: For asthmatics, it has a curative effect. During retention, the air penetrates the bronchioles and activates their linings mildly. As a result of this inner activation, their power is increased and health is restored.

This *asana* has several other benefits. It brings flexibility to the hip joints and corrects disorders of the stomach and intestines. It removes wind and gastric problems of the digestive system.

It tones up the muscles of the sex glands and enhances potency. For women, it cures menstrual disorders. It is easy to do and hence is recommended to all practitioners of yoga.

TARA ASANA
(PALM TREE POSE)

Position of Readiness: Stand up and make a forty-five degree angle with the feet. Let the hands hang loosely at the sides. Keep the body straight and look ahead at eye level. Breathe normally. This is the position of readiness.

Steps of Actual Practice: Before describing the steps, it should be pointed out that this is a *kriya* of the hands and arms. In this *kriya*, the hands are folded six times according to the following process:

(i) Make the hands tight and gradually raise them in front while inhaling. By the time the hands have been brought to the level of the shoulders, inhaling should be completed. Now hold the breath. Turn the palms upward. Keep the hands straight, parallel, and firm. This is the first fold as shown in Figure 22.

(ii) After pausing for a second on the first fold, turn the palms downward and move the hands to their respective sides. During this second fold, let the hands come to the level of the shoulders so that they are in one line. Keep looking straight ahead while holding the breath as shown in Figure 23.

(iii) After pausing for a second on the second fold, bring the hands again in front while keeping the palms downward. Keep the hands tightened and parallel to each other. The distance between them should be six inches for teenagers and eight inches for adults. Pause for a second on this fold.

(iv) Then turn the palms so that they face each other and lift them stiffly towards the sky. The palms should still face each

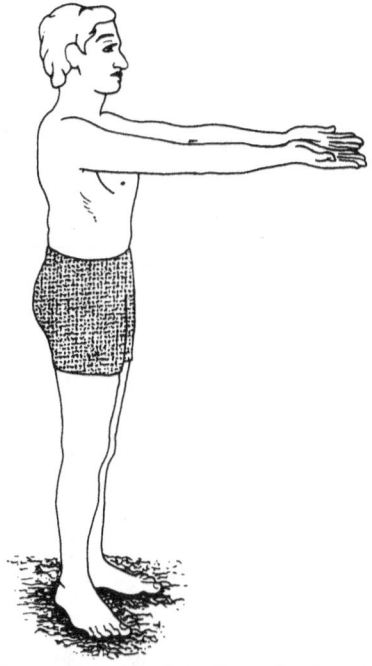

Figure 22. Hands in Front for Tara Asana

other when fully raised and the distance between them should be six to eight inches (Figure 24). Keep looking straight ahead. Do not bend the body. Stay in that position for only a second.

(v) Now turn the palms downward and bring the hands to the sides as they were in the second fold (Figure 23). Palms are down, and the hands are tensed and in a straight line. Stay there for a second. You must retain the breath up to this fold.

(vi) Then start exhaling and slowly lowering the hands. When they have returned to the sides, you should have exhaled completely. Now loosen the body and rest. Let the hands hang loosely. You have completed one round of *Tara asana*. After resting for two deep breaths, make more rounds by following the same process.

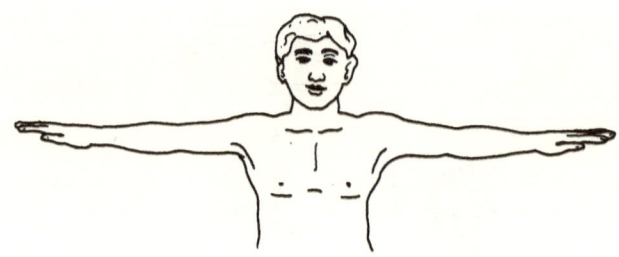

Figure 23. Hands on the Sides in Tara Asana

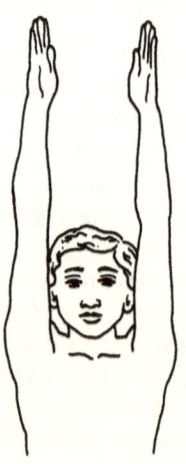

Figure 24. Hands Up in Tara Asana

Daily Practice: Do it only three times a day during the first week. During the second week and after, increase it to four times daily. Five times are the maximum in a day.

Benefits: *Tara asana* strengthens the lungs and chest. Though the outward activation in this *kriya* is of the hands, it internally activates the lungs, muscles of the chest, and the respiratory system. For asthmatics, therefore, it provides a corrective as well as a strengthening effect to their bronchioles and lungs.

For general practitioners, *Tara asana* has several benefits. It enhances the measurement of the chest. Those whose chests are not properly developed can find this *asana* more beneficial by making the chest proportionate. It builds up the chest muscles in an all-round way and has a curative effect for any disorder of this area.

Those who wish to add a few inches to their height might also find it very rewarding. People suffering from pain in their shoulder joints can correct their disorders through *Tara asana*. It is easy to do and can be done by people of any age.

YOGA MUDRA
(YOGA SYMBOL)

Position of Readiness: The perfect way of practicing the *Yoga Mudra* is to be in the Lotus Pose first. But it is not easy for everyone to sit in the Lotus Pose. Hence, those who cannot do it should sit on the floor with folded legs. After being seated either in the Lotus Pose or in *Sukha asana* as shown in Figure 1 and Figure 2, do the following: Bring both hands behind the back. Grab the wrist of one hand with the other hand. Make a fist with the hand which is being held. At this stage, keep the hands loose and let them rest on the back. Straighten the spine. Look in front while keeping the neck and head erect. This is the position of readiness.

Steps of Actual Practice: (i) Exhale gradually and, simultane-

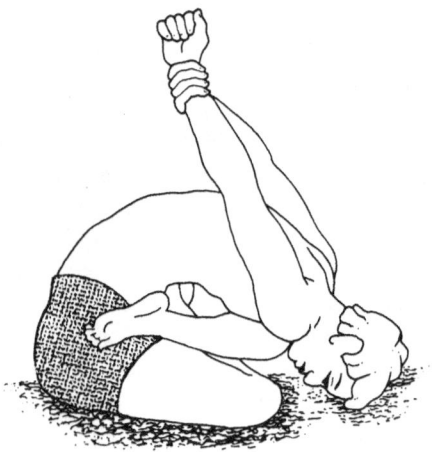

Figure 25.   Yoga Mudra

ously, start lowering the head towards the floor. You have to synchronize exhaling with the bending of the upper part of the body. Let the head come down only as far as it can be lowered easily. Do not put excessive strain on the spine while lowering the head. If possible, touch the ground with the forehead. By the time the head has touched the floor, all air should have been completely exhaled.

(ii) After touching the floor, or only going down as much as possible, retain the breath. Now tighten the hands and gradually raise them (in grabbed form) upwards as high as possible without any excessive strain. Remain in this position for six to eight seconds as shown in Figure 25.

(iii) Start inhaling while lowering the hands and gradually return to the position of readiness. Loosen the hands and the body. Rest for six to eight seconds. After resting, repeat the same process a few more times.

Daily Practice: Only two rounds daily during the first week and increase it to four rounds during the second week. Four rounds are the maximum.

Benefits: It activates and exercises the lungs and their bronchial branches very effectively. Because the upper area of the body is reversed, the blood from the lower region begins to flow upwards and thereby massages the veins of the lower bronchioles of the lungs. This helps restore the normal health of the lungs and their functioning. For these reasons, *Yoga Mudra* has a curative effect for asthmatics.

For general practitioners, *Yoga Mudra* corrects disorders of the spine, removes gastric troubles and constipation, strengthens the digestive system, and enhances sexual potency.

USHTRA ASANA
(CAMEL POSE)

Position of Readiness: You need to have something soft under the knees to do this *asana*. Put a blanket or a towel on the floor and be seated on it. Fold the legs at the knees and keep them about six inches apart. Then kneel and let the ankles and toes of both legs be flat on the floor. Keep the heels about six inches apart. Now the back of the knees, calves, and the heels are in an upward position.

Steps of Actual Practice: (i) Kneel and catch hold of the back

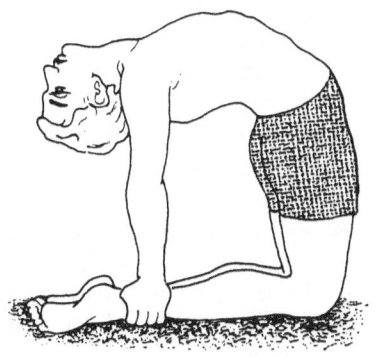

Figure 26. Ushtra Asana

of the ankle of the right leg with the right hand. Hold it firmly. If you cannot reach above the heel, you may just catch the heels.

(ii) Now catch hold of the left heel or the back of the left ankle with the left hand. Make the grip firm.

(iii) Holding the heels or the back of the ankles, straighten the thighs and waist. Bend the head and neck backwards as far as you · can. Push the waist area slightly forward. Breathe normally and stay in that position for six to eight seconds as shown in Figure 26.

(iv) After holding for the desired time, return to the position of readiness by the following process:

Release the left hand first and straighten up the left side of the body a little. Then release the right hand and make the body straight and in the kneeling position. If possible, sit down on the soles and in between the heels and then rest. You have completed one round of *Ushtra asana*.

(v) After resting for six to eight seconds, repeat the same process.

Daily Practice: Only twice daily during the first week. During the second week and afterwards, do it a maximum of four times daily.

Benefits: For asthmatics, *Ushtra asana* has a good effect on the whole respiratory system. This *asana* activates the facial tissues, the nasal passages, the pharynx, the lungs, and all the respiratory organs and nerves. Because of internal as well as external activation during this *asana*, the weakened condition of the respiratory organs is corrected and their normal health is restored.

Ushtra asana has several benefits for the general practitioner. It corrects any disorders of the neck, shoulders, and the spine. It cures various types of vision defects of the eyes and strengthens all the sense organs. People suffering from throat trouble, tonsillitis, voice defects, and chronic headaches will find this *asana* very beneficial. It also conditions the muscles of the chest and makes the chest area proportionate in size. It is not a difficult *asana*; with a little practice, anyone can do it.

SIMHA ASANA
(LION POSE)

Position of Readiness: Put a blanket or a towel on the floor. Bend both legs at the knees and sit on the curve of soles and toes, keeping the heels apart and turned upwards under the hips. Since it might be difficult for some persons to make this curve with the toes, soles, and heels, they are advised to sit on their bent legs in any position they can possibly manage to make.

After being seated either on the curve of the heels or in any position, do the following: straighten the body. Keep the head, neck, and spine in one line. Look in front. Put the palms of the hands on their respective knees. Breathe normally.

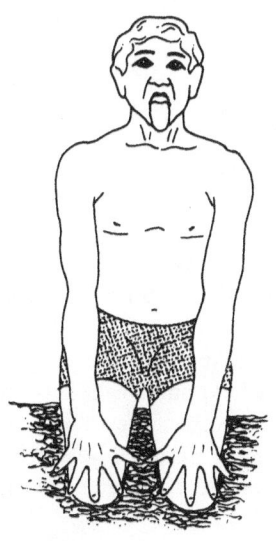

Figure 27. Simha Asana

Steps of Actual Practice: (i) Start exhaling partially through both nostrils and partially through the mouth and, at the same time, start extending the tongue. Do not rush. Protrude the tongue in a straightforward position gradually. Let the tongue come out fully. By the time the tongue has been pushed out, exhalation should be complete. Then hold the breath.

(ii) When the tongue is fully out, spread the fingers of both hands and tighten them. Stretch the eyes and make them look frightening. Keep the whole body tense. Stay in this tight and strained condition for about six to eight seconds. You are in the *Simha asana* as shown in Figure 27.

(iii) After holding the *asana* for a few seconds, start inhaling and withdrawing the tongue. Loosen the body gradually while inhaling and pulling back the tongue. When the tongue has been fully withdrawn, close the mouth and breathe normally and rest for a few seconds. Relax the whole body while remaining seated in the same position.

(iv) After resting for six to eight seconds, repeat the same process a few more times.

Daily Practice: Begin with two rounds daily during the first week. From the second week onward, do four rounds daily. Do not make more than four rounds in a single sitting. In certain cases, this *asana* can be performed twice daily after letting eight hours elapse between the first and the second sitting.

Benefits: *Simha asana* is very famous for its various remarkable benefits. It has medicinal value for curing throat trouble, voice deficiency, and tonsillitis.

It also has a good effect on the respiratory system. It activates the larynx, trachea, and all the bronchioles. It invigorates the thyroid cartilages. Because of this internal activation and invigoration, health is restored to the whole respiratory system and its disorders are removed. This is an easy *asana* which can be done by anyone.

SARVANGA ASANA
(WHOLE BODY POSE)

Position of Readiness: Lie down on your back on the floor. Place the palms down next to the body. Bring the heels and toes together and keep them loose. Straighten the whole body and look towards the ceiling. Breathe normally.

Steps of Actual Practice: (i) Stretch out the toes of both legs and tighten them. Then start inhaling and, at the same time, start lifting both legs together towards the ceiling. Inhale in such a way that, by the time the legs have been brought to a perpendicular position, the inhalation is complete.

(ii) When the inhaling is completed and both legs are fully upward, bring both the palms under the hips and raise the whole body upward by pushing it with both hands while

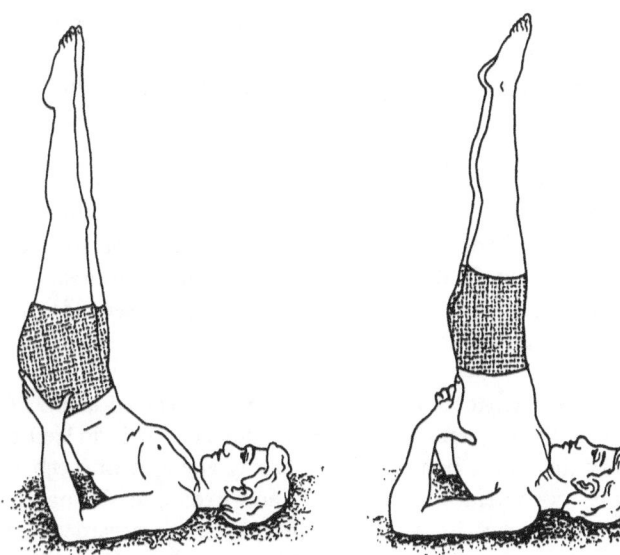

Figure 28.   Half Sarvanga Asana   Figure 29.   Sarvanga Asana

exhaling. During this second stage, do the following: Raise the body upward gradually. Let the hands help to push up the body. Do not try to raise the body with any excessive strain. Go only as high as your body permits (Figure 28). Keep both palms on both sides of the back for support. When the body has been raised to the maximum (as shown in Figure 29), stay there and breathe normally. Tighten the legs and keep them together. Stay in this position for ten to fifteen seconds during the first week. Gradually increase the time to one minute in a month and up to three minutes during the second month.

(iii) After standing on the shoulders for the desired time, return to the floor by the following method: Bend the legs at the knees first. This will bring the heels onto the hips. Gradually move the palms towards the hips and let the body come down slowly to the floor. While returning, support the body's weight with the hands. Make it a smooth return. When the hips touch the floor, drop the heels down near the hips first. Put the palms on the floor on both sides of the body. Then stretch out the legs and let them fall on the floor. You have made one round of *Sarvanga asana*.

(iv) Rest for about ten seconds; while resting, breathe normally.

Daily Practice: *Sarvanga asana* is done only once. It is not a repeatable *asana*. The difference lies in the length of time the posture is held. Those who have practiced this *asana* for more than a month can hold it for three minutes—the *maximum* time for holding it. Beginners should start it with ten seconds only and should increase the time gradually.

Benefits: *Sarvanga asana* is one of the most valued *asanas* of the Hatha Yoga system. As its name indicates, it is indeed an *asana* of the whole body. There is hardly any area of the body which is not energized, activated, and exercised during this *asana*. Because of its wholeness in effect, it is regarded next only to the king of all *asanas*—*Shirsha asana* (Head Stand Pose).

For asthmatics, *Sarvanga asana* has therapeutic value. It exercises all the bronchioles and the lungs completely. Since the whole respiratory system is invigorated and strengthened during this *asana*, lung troubles are corrected.

The *asana* has countless benefits. Therefore it is a very desirable *asana* for general practitioners. It corrects any disorder of the circulatory system; supplies blood to the facial tissues; removes constipation, gastric disorders, and abdominal troubles; strengthens the digestive system; and energizes all the sex glands.

MATSYA ASANA
(FISH POSE)

After practicing *Sarvanga asana*, it is necessary to do *Matsya asana*. There are several good reasons for this. Certain *asanas* activate certain parts of the body more than others. To reverse this difference of impact, such *asanas* are followed by particular *asanas* to create a balance. For example, during *Sarvanga asana* the head, neck, and shoulders are passive and the lower areas of the body are active. To create a balance, *Sarvanga* is followed by the *Matsya asana* so that the head, neck, and shoulders become active and the lower areas of the body remain passive. Thus, by doing the *Matsya asana* after the *Sarvanga asana*, the whole body is activated properly and in a balanced way.

There are two ways of doing the *Matsya asana*:

(i) With the Lotus Pose, and (ii) without being in the Lotus Pose.

Though the first form is regarded as superior to the second, basically both are equally beneficial. Since it is not possible for everyone to make the Lotus Pose, both forms are described so that every person can practice this *asana*.

Position of Readiness: Be in any one of the following two positions:

(i) Sit in the Lotus Pose. Then lie down on your back while

keeping the legs folded in the Lotus form. After the spine, neck, and head are resting on the floor completely, lower the thighs. Put the hands on the floor next to the body. Keep the palms down. Breathe normally. This is the position of readiness with the Lotus Pose. If you cannot do this, try the second method described below;

(ii) Lie down on the floor on your back. Bend the legs at the knees and bring the heels near the hips. Keep the knees together and the heels separated from each other by about four inches. Put the palms on the floor. Straighten the body. Look upward and breathe normally. This is the easy way of readiness.

Steps of Actual Practice: Bring the palms under the thighs. Then, while pulling on the thighs, lift the head slightly upward. Let the weight of the upper part of the body rest on the elbows. Then bend the head backward and make an arch by bending the backbone. After the arch (curve) has been made, rest the head on the floor. To make a bigger arch, give more pull on the thighs and more twist on the neck and back. But do not pull

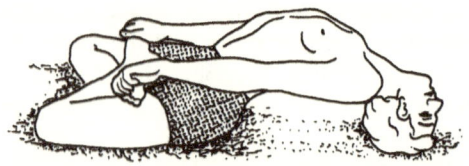

Figure 30. Matsya Asana with Lotus Pose

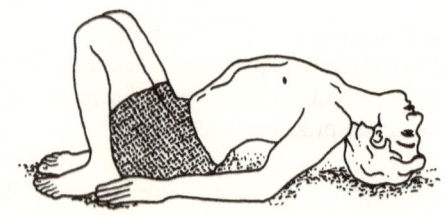

Figure 31. Easy Matsya Asana

excessively. In the beginning, start with a minimum amount of stretching.

(ii) When the arch has been made according to the capability of your body's condition, stay in that position. If your arch is in the Lotus Pose, then grab the toes of the left leg with the right hand and those of the right leg with the left hand and give a light pull on them as shown in Figure 30. If you are doing the *Matsya asana* the easy way, without the Lotus Pose, then stretch out both hands alongside the body and keep the palms on the floor as shown in Figure 31.

(iii) Now take a few deep but slow and gradual breaths. Stay in this position for about six to eight seconds. This completes the *Matsya asana*.

(iv) After being in *Matsya asana* for the desired period, return to the position of readiness by the following process: If you were holding the toes, release them and bring the palms down on the floor. Then pull the thighs with your hands again by bending the elbows. Now lift the head upwards and straighten the neck and head. Gradually bring the back, shoulders, neck, and head to the floor, unfold the legs and stretch them on the floor, and rest.

(v) Rest for two to three normal breaths. After the rest is over, make one or two more rounds by following the same process.

Daily Practice: Two to four times daily.

Benefits: For asthmatics, *Matsya asana* corrects disorders of the whole respiratory system. This is because all the organs concerned with respiration, such as the nasal passages, the pharynx, the larynx, the trachea, the bronchi, and the lungs, are well exercised during this *asana*.

Matsya asana provides several other benefits. It has a good effect on the facial tissues. It activates the spine and all the muscles of the back. Because of this activation, disorders of the spine and back are corrected. It removes stiffness of the neck and back, and brings flexibility to the whole upper area of the body. It corrects their malfunctioning.

Its easy form can be practiced by any person of any age. Since it is a highly beneficial *asana*, it is recommended to all yoga practitioners.

CHAPTER 5

Arthritis

ARTHRITIS is a disease of the joints. People suffering from this disease have a burning feeling, terrible pain, and aching in their affected joints. There is swelling, redness, stiffness, and heat in the joints. There are several variations of arthritis; the most common are rheumatoid arthritis, gout, and osteoarthritis.

It is difficult to explain the root cause of all these kinds of arthritis because there are various reasons for it. For example, it could be due to an improper diet, lack of proper exercise, lack of hygiene, poor health, and other similar factors.

Millions of people suffer from this vexing, torturous, and sometimes crippling disease. It affects men and women of all ages. The most disheartening aspect of the disease is that it is not easily cured through medicine when it is chronic.

It is a common practice all over the world to prescribe medicines and recommend physical exercises to cure this disease. Since Therapeutic Yoga is not yet well known to medical practitioners, they do not make use of it to treat arthritis.

In treating arthritic patients at our Institute in India, we have found that a regular practice of some selected yoga *asanas* cures this disease within two months when the arthritis is moderate. In chronic cases, it takes four to five months or even longer to restore normal health. The most remarkable aspect of yoga treatment is that it cures the disease permanently without the use of any medicine.

Treatment

Arthritic or rheumatic patients must do three things: (i) practice selected yoga *asanas* regularly, (ii) eat a proper diet, and (iii) maintain proper hygienic care. A detailed description of these aspects is given below:

(i) **Yoga Asanas:** Arthritics are advised to practice *Santulan asana, Trikona asana, Veera asana, Gomukha asana, Vriksha asana, Setubandha asana, Siddha asana, Natraj asana,* and *Shava asana.* The method of practicing each of these *asanas* is presented in the following pages. A regular practice of these *asanas* will cure any type of arthritis without the use of any medicine. Those who take medicine are advised to stop it after they have practiced yoga for two to three weeks.

(ii) **Proper Diet:** A proper diet is essential for arthritic or rheumatic people. Therefore, they are advised to stop eating bananas and yogurt. Those who smoke or take tobacco in any form should stop it completely or reduce its intake considerably. No more than two cups of coffee or tea should be taken within twenty-four hours.

They should eat four times daily. For breakfast, they should eat an orange, apple, or any fruit (except bananas), germinated chick-peas, and whole wheat bread. They can take a cup of hot milk with Ovaltine. Non-vegetarians may have a boiled or poached egg. For lunch and dinner, they should first take salad (a mixture of tomato, carrot, cucumber, radish, lettuce, or any eatable raw vegetables). After eating about a cup of salad, they should eat soup, wheat bread, and green vegetables. Non-vegetarians can eat fish and liver with the least amount of spices. Patients should avoid the excessive use of hot spices, drink ten to twelve glasses of fresh water daily, and eat at least two hours before retiring for the night.

In the afternoon, they should take some light refreshment, such as fresh fruit, salted crackers, or cake.

(iii) **Hygienic Care:** It is important to bathe regularly, keep the whole body clean, and take proper care of the teeth. The bath can be taken with hot or cold water, as desired. The whole body should be thoroughly rubbed with a rough soapy wash-cloth. To derive the full benefits from water, rubbing the whole body is essential.

It is also important to wear clean clothes. Neatness and cleanliness should be maintained daily as much as possible.

If arthritics follow the above-mentioned system of yoga therapy, they should feel assured of getting fully cured from this disease. They are advised to begin their practice according to the method described in this chapter. During the first week, they should practice only two to four *asanas* of this series. After practicing the desired number of *asanas*, they are advised to do the *Shava asana* as described in Chapter 2. Your daily yoga practice should be completed by doing *Shava asana* at the end. *Shava asana* should be done for one-fourth of the total time spent for practicing yoga.

During the second week and after, they should gradually add other *asanas*. They should never try to do all the *asanas* of this series during the first week.

SANTULAN ASANA
(BALANCING POSE)

Position of Readiness: Place a carpet, blanket, or mat on the floor and stand on it. Make the body straight and firm. Look straight ahead. Let the hands hang at the sides. This is the position of readiness.

Note: To do this *asana*, you will have to stand on one leg at a time. It is not easy for everyone to do so. Therefore, those who might have any difficulty in standing on one leg on the floor should stand near a wall to support the body's weight.

Steps of Actual Practice: (i) Stand up on the right leg and bend the left leg at the knee. Bring the heel of the left leg near the hip. If the heel cannot be brought to the hip due to pain in the knee, bend the leg backward as much as possible.

(ii) Catch the toes of the left leg with the left hand so that all the toes are held in the palm. Bring the heel of the folded leg to the hip or close to it.

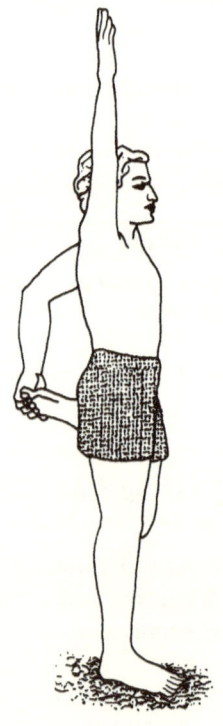

Figure 32.   Santulan Asana

(iii) Tighten the right arm. Keep all the fingers together and slowly raise the right arm above the head. Do not rush in lifting. Keep the palm facing downwards while raising the hand. When the hand is fully raised, the palm should be straight and face forward.

(iv) Hold this position for six to eight seconds, keeping the lifted arm tight and firm. The right leg on which you are standing should be tight and straight. Keep looking straight ahead. There is no special breathing requirement for this *asana*; breathe normally while doing it (as shown in Figure 32).

(v) After staying in this position for six to eight seconds, return to the position of readiness in the following manner: Slowly lower the lifted arm, still keeping it stiff. Do not drop it. When the raised hand has reached the side, release the left leg and slowly lower it to the floor. You are now in the position of readiness again after completing one round of *Santulan asana.*

After resting for six seconds, stand on the left leg and bend the right leg and raise the left hand in the same way as you did the first time. Make further rounds alternately by following the same process.

Daily Practice: Only four times daily during the first week. After a week, increase it to six times a day.

Benefits: *Santulan asana* is mainly a *kriya* of the major joints of the body. It removes their rigidity and makes them flexible. It also normalizes the blood circulation in the affected areas and tones up the muscles. As a result of enhanced blood circulation and muscle conditioning, pain in the joints is corrected.

This *asana* has a curative effect on the knees, ankles, shoulder joints, wrists, palms, and fingers. It is an easy *asana* and any person can do it either standing on the floor or with the help of the wall. For general yoga practitioners, it is a good *asana* for activating their bodies and making their joints flexible.

TRIKONA ASANA
(TRIANGLE POSE)

Position of Readiness: Stand with the legs about two and one-half feet apart. Look in front. Let the hands hang loosely at the sides. Make the legs firm and tight.

Steps of Actual Practice: (i) Inhale slowly and at the same time raise both arms up to shoulder level. Keep the hands stiff while raising them. This will bring both arms in one line. The palms should be facing downwards. By the time the hands have come up to shoulder level, inhaling should be completed. Stay there for two seconds. You should be as shown in Figure 33.

(ii) Start exhaling and simultaneously lower the left hand to

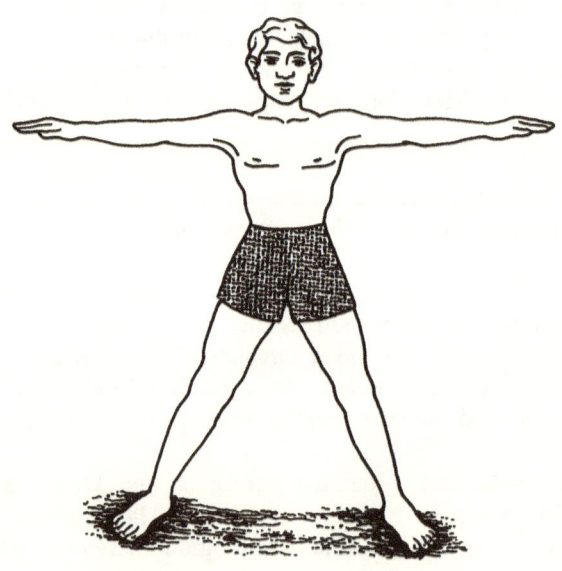

Figure 33. First Phase of Trikona Asana

touch the left foot and raise the right hand up towards the sky. By the time you have touched the foot, you should have completed exhaling. Now hold the breath.

While going down, bend forward, not sideways. Keep looking at the toes you are going to touch. Try to touch the toes of the left foot. After touching them, turn your head right and raise it towards the sky. Now try to see the palm of the right hand. At this point your hands are again in one line. Keep looking at the right palm for about two seconds. Do not bend your legs. Keep the legs quite tight. See Figure 34 for this second phase.

(iii) After looking at the right palm for a few seconds, stretch the upper hand tightly in front of you and look at the floor

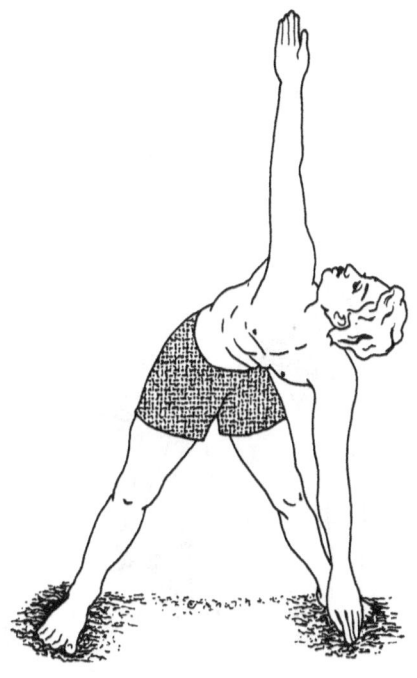

Figure 34. Second Phase of Trikona Asana

beneath that palm. During this stage, your left hand remains on the toes of the left foot and your right hand is fully stretched out in front of you. Your body is bent right in front and the legs are firm and tight. The right arm is close to the right temple. Keep holding the breath. Your posture is as shown in Figure 35.

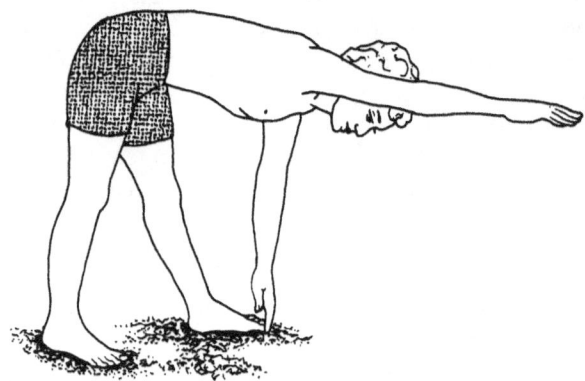

Figure 35. Third Phase of Trikona Asana

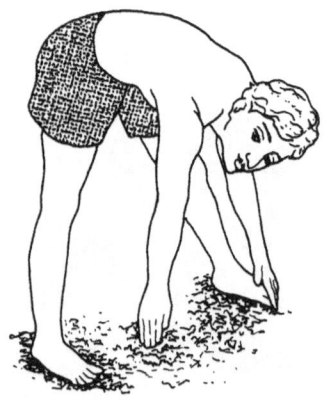

Figure 36. Final Phase of Trikona Asana

(iv) Then turn the right hand forty-five degrees to the right side while keeping the arm and the hand stretched out. At this stage, the fingers of the right hand are together and the palm is about one foot above the ground. Look at the ground where the fingers of the right hand are pointing, as shown in Figure 36. Stay in this position for two seconds. Keep holding the breath.

Now place the right hand on the right leg and start inhaling and standing up. While coming up, drag your hands lightly on the legs until you are back in the standing position. After returning to the position of readiness, your hands are again at the sides. Your have completed one round of *Trikona asana*. Now rest for two normal breaths.

(v) After resting for about five seconds, repeat the *asana* by following the same process. In the second round you have to touch the right foot and raise the left hand towards the sky. Make further rounds alternately.

Daily Practice: Four alternate rounds daily during the first week. During the second week and afterwards, make six rounds daily. Never do more than eight rounds in a single day.

Benefits: *Trikona asana* has medicinal value for curing the pain or any disorder of the neck and the shoulder joints. People suffering from stiffness in the neck will find this *asana* very effective in correcting that disorder.

This *asana* has a good effect on the spine, hip joints, hands, and the palms. All the major joints above the waist are properly activated and their muscles are duly toned up by this *asana*. Arthritics are advised to practice *Santulan asana* first and then the *Trikona asana*. By doing them one after the other, all major and minor joints of the body are fully activated and their functioning is normalized.

For general practitioners, *Trikona asana* has several good benefits. It develops the power of vision, brings flexibility to the spine, and increases mental attentiveness. It is an easy *asana* and hence is recommended to all practitioners of yoga.

VEERA ASANA
(BRAVE POSE)

Position of Readiness: Be seated on the floor in an easy way. Keep the body straight upward. Look ahead at eye level and breathe normally.

Steps of Actual Practice: (i) Bend one leg at the knee and bring its heel behind the hips. The toes of this leg should be on the floor. The heel is up, touching the hip. There is no body weight on the folded leg, all the weight of the body is on the floor.

(ii) Now bend the other leg at the knee and bring this foot onto the thigh of the folded leg. Let the knee of this leg fall on the floor and let its sole rest on the thigh of the other leg.

(iii) Stretch both hands on their respective sides and place the wrists on the top of the head. Then let the palms and fingers of

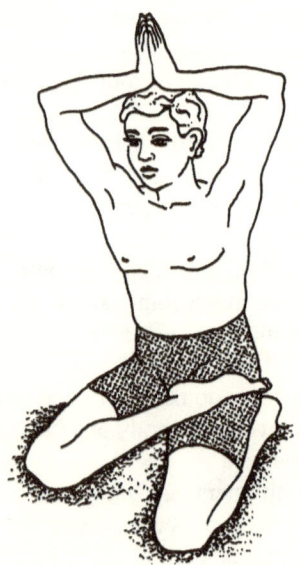

Figure 37.   Veera Asana

both hands touch. Keep the wrists on top of the head and keep the fingers straight up. Then try to straighten the elbows on their respective sides as much as is comfortably possible.

(iv) Now straighten the spine, neck, and the head. Look in front. Keep the palms and fingers together. Your elbows should remain straight and tight. Keep breathing normally. You are in *Veera asana*. Stay in this position for eight seconds, as shown in Figure 37.

(v) After eight seconds, unfold the palms and lower the hands. Then lift the upper foot with the hand and bring it down on the floor. Pull back the other bent leg and bring it to an easy pose. Now rest for five seconds. You have completed one round of *Veera asana*. Do more rounds alternately. During the second round, the leg which was up will be folded backward and the other foot will be put on its thigh.

Daily Practice: Four rounds daily. It might be increased to a maximum of six rounds. Do not practice more than six rounds in a single day.

Benefits: *Veera asana* exercises all the major and minor joints very effectively in a single process. The external activation enhances the blood circulation in the joints and restores their normal health.

The *asana* also strengthens the lungs and the chest. It tones up the muscles of the thighs, hips, and the arms, and eliminates the fat from these areas.

It has also a symbolic value. It is held that those practicing *Veera asana* will develop courage, boldness, and bravery.

GOMUKHA ASANA
(COW HEAD POSE)

Position of Readiness: The proper position of readiness for *Gomukha asana* might be difficult for those arthritics whose knees, ankles, and toes are severely affected. Therefore, these patients are advised to sit on the floor by simply bending the legs at the knees and keeping the spine straight.

Those who can make the proper position of readiness should sit on the floor according to the following steps: Kneel on the floor and keep the body's weight on both knees. Keep the knees separated by about four inches. Let the ankles and toes of both legs rest on the floor so that the toes are close to each other but the heels are upwards, spread out.

This will make an arch-like curve with the toes, soles, and the heels. Gradually sit down on the curve of the soles and place the weight of the whole body on it. Put the palms on the thighs. Look in front at eye level. Keep the spine quite straight. You are now in the perfect position of readiness for *Gomukha asana*, as shown in Figure 15.

Steps of Actual Practice: (i) Slowly bring the right hand to the back. Bend it at the elbow and then raise the back of the hand up towards the neck. This will keep the back of the palm pressed against the spine. Let the fingers of the right hand face upwards. Keep the right hand firmly in that position.

(ii) Now bend your left hand at the elbow, raise it upward, and place the left palm on the left shoulder. Then, first try to touch the fingers of the left hand with the right hand. Some people might have difficulty in even touching the fingers. They should make the move as much as possible and then stay there. Those who do not have any difficulty in touching the fingers should make a lock by folding the fingers of both the hands. To make the lock, the fingers are slightly crooked and then these crooks may be hooked together and pulled against each other.

(iii) After locking the fingers of both hands, try to raise the elbow of the left hand straight upward. Keep the spine firm and straight. Look in front. Breathe normally. Stay in this locked position for six to eight seconds. Those who cannot make the lock should attempt to attain this position as much as is possible and should then stay there for six to eight seconds in the same position. When the fingers of one hand are locked against the fingers of the other hand in that sitting position, the

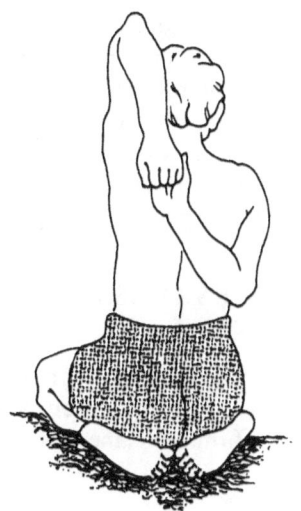

Figure 38.   Gomukha Asana

Gomukha asana is perfectly completed as shown in Figure 38.

(iv) After remaining in this position for six to eight seconds, loosen the grip on the fingers and unlock them gradually. Then slowly bring both hands onto the thighs and rest. You have made one round of *Gomukha asana*. After resting for two normal breaths, make more rounds alternately by following the same process. This means that you must now bring the left hand on the back and raise the elbow of the right hand.

Daily Practice: Four rounds daily during the first week. During the second week and afterward, make six rounds daily. Do it alternately.

Benefits: *Gomukha asana* has, as a single exercise, a corrective effect on all the major and minor joints of the body. It exercises the finger joints, elbows, shoulder joints, toes, ankles, the knees, and the hip joints very effectively. All the muscles and nerves related to various joints are automatically toned up, activated, and normalized.

Because the muscles of the joints are activated, blood circulation is improved in them. As a result, waste products are removed from the joints. It restores the synovial fluid (joint fluid) and thereby removes spasticity and pain.

For general practitioners, this *asana* brings flexibility to the joints, strengthens the bones, increases the measurement of the chest, and enhances the strength of the lungs and heart.

VRIKSHA ASANA
(TREE POSE)

Position of Readiness: Stand on the floor and look in front at eye level. Keep the hands hanging loosely at the sides. Make the body straight and firm. Breathe normally. This is the position of readiness.

Steps of Actual Practice: You have to stand on one leg in this *asana*. If you have difficulty in standing on one leg, use a wall or a pillar for support. Then do the following:

(i) Stand on the left leg and fold back the right leg at the knee. Bring the right foot onto the thigh of the left leg so that the outer part of the heel and sole rest on it. This will twist the right foot a little and press its side against the left thigh. Do not press the thigh with the heel itself, but with its side. When the side of the heel has been pressed firmly against the left thigh, make the left leg and the whole body tight and straight.

(ii) Then raise both hands sideways towards the head. When the hands are stretched above the head, join the palms and the fingers. Then bring the palms to the head so that the wrists rest on it.

(iii) After the palms have been placed on the head, you must do several things: Try to pull the folded elbows backward to bring them in one line. But do not exert too much. Look straight forward at eye level. Tighten the leg you are standing on. Now, the whole body is tight. Breathe normally. Stay in that position for six to eight seconds. You are in *Vriksha asana*, as shown in Figure 39.

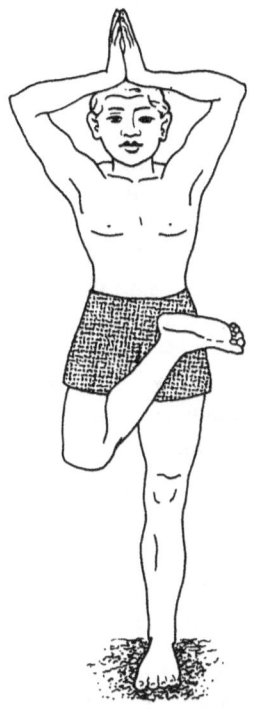

Figure 39. Vriksha Asana

(iv) After holding that *asana* for the desired time, loosen the pressure on the palms and stretch out the arms in order to bring them back tightly to their respective sides. When the hands are at the sides, grab the toes of the folded leg, lift it slightly upwards, and then drop it to the floor. You are now back in the position of readiness. Rest for two normal breaths.

(v) After resting for a few seconds, repeat the *asana* a few more times, alternating the legs. For example, in the second round you must stand on the right leg and fold the left one. Then follow the steps done in the first round to complete this *asana*.

Daily Practice: Four rounds daily during the first week. During the second week and afterwards, make six rounds daily. Keep alternating the legs when making further rounds. Do not do more than six rounds in a single day.

Benefits: *Vriksha asana* activates all the joints of the body. All the major and minor joints of the body are affected by this single *asana*. It tones up the muscles of the ankles, toes, knees, hip and shoulder joints, elbows, hands, and fingers. As a result of this activation and conditioning of the joint muscles, blood circulation becomes normal in the joints and they regain strength.

For general practitioners, *Vriksha asana* conditions and strengthens their bodily joints and bones. It brings flexibility to the legs and hands and enhances the measurement of the chest. It is an easy *asana* and hence every practitioner of yoga can do it.

SETUBANDHA ASANA
(BRIDGE POSE)

Position of Readiness: Lie down with your back on the floor. Bend the legs at the knees and bring the heels close to the hips. Keep the heels about two to three inches apart. Let the knees also be about three inches apart. Bring your hands close to the

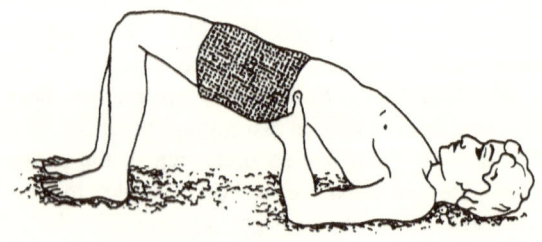

Figure 40.   Setubandha Asana

body on both sides. Put the palms on the floor. Look straight up and breathe normally. This is the position of readiness.

Steps of Actual Practice: (i) Lift the hips and waist up while keeping the shoulders and feet on the floor. When the hips have been raised, support them with the palms on both sides.

(ii) Gradually keep raising the hips upwards while pushing the palms towards the waist. Let the hands help raise the waist up as high as it can be raised without strain. Now support the body's weight on the thumbs and the index fingers and the palms on the sides. Let the shoulders, neck, and head remain firmly on the floor. Try to be sure that the thighs are parallel to one another with a gap of about three inches. Keep breathing normally. Stay in this position for six to eight seconds, as shown in Figure 40.

(iii) After remaining in the raised position for six to eight seconds, start lowering the hips toward the floor while still supporting the body with the palms. Do not let the body drop on the floor; bring it down slowly. When the hips, waist, and the back are on the floor, place your palms on the floor on both sides of the body. Stretch out the legs on the floor and rest for two to three normal breaths.

(iv) After resting for a few seconds, repeat the *asana* by following the same process as you did during the first round.

Daily Practice: Four rounds daily during the first week. During the second week and afterwards, do a maximum of six rounds. Do not ever make more than six rounds in a single day.

Benefits: The main impact of *Setubandha asana* is on the spine and the hip joints. Those who have pain either in any part of the spine or in the hip joints are strongly advised to practice this *asana*. It also relieves pain and corrects disorders of the shoulder joints, neck, arms, and the palms. Since it is an easy *asana*, arthritics in any condition and of any age can do it.

For general practitioners, it is a good *asana* for making the spine flexible, for removing wind and gastric troubles, and for correcting respiratory disorders.

SIDDHA ASANA
(AUSPICIOUS POSE)

Persons with moderate joint pain of any type can be completely cured if they practice the *asanas* of this series described above. Chronic cases, however, might take a little longer time than up to this point to become fully cured. Therefore, patients with chronic arthritis are advised to practice all the *asanas* of this series regularly. By continuing the practice, they should be fully cured in four to six months.

It must be emphasized that one must eat a proper diet along with the regular practice of yoga to get satisfactory results. The diet for arthritics has been fully described in the first part of this chapter. It is expected that they take their meals according to what I have recommended. I wish only to remind them again not to eat yogurt and bananas, and to avoid taking tea, coffee, and cigarettes on an empty stomach. With these clarifications, a new *asana—Siddha asana—*is presented now.

Position of Readiness: Sit on a carpeted floor and stretch out both legs in front. Keep your spine straight and firm. Look in front. Keep the hands on the floor. Breathe normally. This is the position of readiness.

Steps of Actual Practice: (i) Bend the left leg at the knee and bring the foot toward you. Stretch the toes and ankle of the left leg and try to bring them in a straight line. If you find it difficult to bring them in a straight line, stretch them only as much as possible. Bring the heel near the genitals without pressing against them. Your left knee should now be on the floor. If the knee cannot touch the floor, let it remain a little up and raised.

(ii) Now bend the right leg at the knee and bring the right

foot on top of the left foot. Keep the right heel just above the left heel. Then stretch the toes and ankle of the right leg while keeping the right knee also on the floor. Keep the legs in the same position. Do not put any pressure on the genitals.

(iii) Stretch out both hands. Make a circle with the thumb and index finger of each hand and keep them firmly together. Now put the right wrist on the right knee and the left wrist on the left knee. Make the arms and hands tight. Keep the spine straight and firm. Your head, neck, and spine should be in one line. Your fingers should be pointing towards the earth. Keep looking ahead at eye level. Breathe normally. Now you are in *Siddha asana*, as shown in Figure 41.

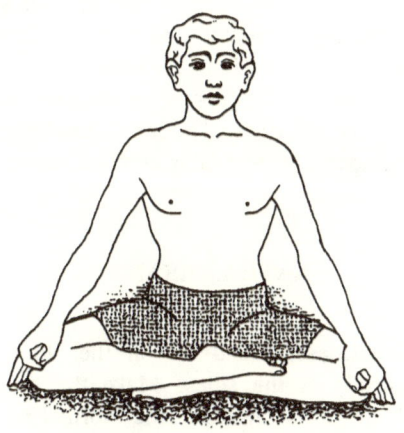

Figure 41. Siddha Asana

(iv) Stay in this position for about one minute and then loosen the fingers of both hands. Lift the right leg by hand and place it on the floor and stretch out the legs. After resting for a few seconds, repeat the *asana* once more by alternating the legs. This time your right foot will be underneath and the left foot will be on top. Stay in this *asana* again for about a minute.

Daily Practice: Practice *Siddha asana* for a maximum of three minutes only. Begin with about two minutes and gradually increase the time to three minutes daily. During this period, you will be doing *Siddha asana* only twice and the total time spent will be three minutes only. Do not practice it for more than three minutes in one day.

Benefits: *Siddha asana* has a good curative effect on all the joints below the waist. The hip joints, knees, and ankles are very effectively activated during this *asana* and, as a result, the circulation of blood in these areas becomes normalized, the supply of synovial fluid (joint fluid) is restored, and the spasticity and pain are removed.

Siddha asana has a good effect on the nervous system of the body. People suffering from any kind of nerve defects will find this *asana* very beneficial. It is regarded as a vitally important *asana* for gaining the power of concentration and for acquiring mental equilibrium. Though it might appear a little difficult for beginners, with regular practice, any person can do it properly.

NATRAJ ASANA
(ACTION POSE)

Position of Readiness: Stand up on the floor and let the hands hang loosely at the sides. Make the body tense and straight. Look in front and breathe normally. This is the position of readiness.

Steps of Actual Practice: (i) Stand on the left leg. Bend the right leg back at the knee. Grab all the toes of the right leg with the palm of the right hand. At this stage, your right leg is bent backwards and is held by the palm. Keep the leg in the same position.

(ii) Now bring all the fingers of the left hand together and tighten the left hand. When you have done this, slowly raise this hand up and at the same time slowly push the right leg backwards. In this process, you are doing two things simultaneously: You are raising the left hand in front and pushing the right foot backwards. While doing this, you should give a maximum backward push with the right leg. But do not raise the left hand straight up; keep it slanted and pointed towards the horizon, so that the whole hand is visible to you.

(iii) Now bend the body slightly forward above the waist and try to see the top of the fingers of the left hand and keep looking there. Keep the right foot fully pushed back and tight. Make the left leg quite firm and tight. Do not loosen the left leg when you bend the body slightly forward. Stay in this position for about eight seconds, as shown in Figure 42. Keep breathing normally during this *asana*. If you have difficulty in doing this *asana* standing, use either a wall or a pillar for support. After you have become used to practicing it this way, do it standing, without any support.

(iv) After remaining in this position for about eight seconds,

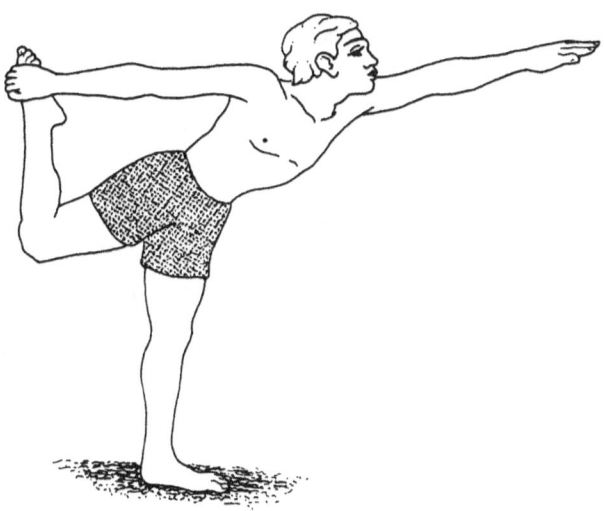

Figure 42.   Natraj Asana

gradually bring the left hand tightly down and bring the right leg back to the folded position and then release it. You are now standing on both legs. Rest in this position for a few seconds and then repeat the *asana*. This time, stand up on the right leg, hold the left leg, and raise the right hand. You must do it alternately by following the same process as during the first round.

Daily Practice: Four rounds daily during the first week. During the second week and afterwards, make six rounds daily. Practice it alternately. Do not do more than six rounds of *Natraj asana* in a single day.

Benefits: *Natraj asana* activates all the major and minor joints of the body in a single process. For arthritics, it has a great curative effect upon all the joints. It properly activates the shoulder and hip joints, the knees, ankles, palms, and the fingers. Because of this conditioning, the muscles, nerves, and tissues of these areas become normal and their functioning is restored.

Natraj asana also has a good effect on the spine: It removes spinal rigidity, pain, backache, stiffness, and other disorders of the spine.

To general practitioners, it provides flexibility to the limbs, strengthens the major bones, enhances digestive power, improves eyesight, and generates vitality, potency, and the quality of determination. A significant aspect of *Natraj asana* is that it symbolizes action. In other words, it breaks the condition of standing still in an individual and creates a feeling of action. Because of these benefits, it is a highly recommended *asana* for arthritics as well as for the general practitioners of yoga.

CHAPTER 6

Obesity

OBESITY is a worldwide health hazard. Millions of people of every age are carrying excessive weight on their bodies. The most frightening aspect of obesity is that it shortens the life span; causes arteriosclerosis, coronary heart troubles, hypertension (high blood pressure), various physical-mental (psychosomatic) ailments and disorders; and makes the life of the person miserable because complications develop such as diabetes, indigestion, gastrointestinal disorders, sexual incapacitation, and an inferiority complex.

To better understand the problems related to obesity, we must differentiate it from overweight. Overweight is not obesity; but every obese person is overweight. Being overweight means carrying only a few pounds of extra weight than the body frame requires. In case of overweight, though there is unwanted and extra weight, it may not be quite excessive. For example, if an adult of average height carries five to ten pounds of extra weight, he is overweight but not obese.

Unlike one who is overweight, the obese person's weight

AVERAGE WEIGHT FOR MEN AND WOMEN

MEN

Weight without wearing shoes and heavy clothes.

Weight in lbs. according to age

Feet	Inches	15 to 19 yrs	20 to 24 yrs	25 to 29 yrs	30 to 34 yrs	35 to 39 yrs	40 to 44 yrs	45 to 49 yrs	50 to 54 yrs	55 to 59 yrs
5	0	113	119	124	127	129	132	134	135	136
5	1	115	121	126	129	131	134	136	137	138
5	2	118	124	128	131	133	136	138	139	140
5	3	121	127	131	134	136	139	141	142	143
5	4	124	131	134	137	140	142	144	145	146
5	5	128	135	138	141	144	146	148	149	150
5	6	132	139	142	145	148	150	152	153	154
5	7	136	142	146	149	152	154	156	157	158
5	8	140	146	150	154	157	159	161	162	163
5	9	144	150	154	158	162	164	166	167	168
5	10	148	154	158	163	167	169	171	172	173
5	11	153	158	163	168	172	175	177	178	179
6	0	158	163	169	174	178	181	183	184	185
6	1	163	168	175	180	184	187	190	191	192
6	2	168	173	181	186	191	194	197	198	199

WOMEN

Weight without wearing shoes and heavy clothes.

Weight in lbs. according to age

Feet	Inches	15 to 19 yrs	20 to 24 yrs	25 to 29 yrs	30 to 34 yrs	35 to 39 yrs	40 to 44 yrs	45 to 49 yrs	50 to 54 yrs	55 to 59 yrs
5	0	108	115	118	121	124	128	131	133	134
5	1	110	117	120	123	126	130	133	135	137
5	2	113	120	122	125	129	133	136	138	140
5	3	116	123	125	128	132	136	139	141	143
5	4	119	126	129	132	136	139	142	144	146
5	5	122	129	132	136	140	143	146	148	150
5	6	126	133	136	140	144	147	151	152	153
5	7	130	137	140	144	148	151	155	157	158
5	8	134	141	144	148	152	155	159	162	163
5	9	138	145	148	152	156	159	163	166	167
5	10	142	149	152	155	159	162	166	170	173
5	11	147	153	155	158	162	166	170	174	177
6	0	150	157	159	162	165	169	173	177	182

becomes almost static. Any adult of average height carrying more than ten extra pounds for years is obese. This excessive weight begins to strain all the bodily organs constantly and, as a consequence, the individual faces health hazards. The preceding charts show what the average weight of men and women should be.

Though obesity causes the same disproportionate accumulation of fat in men and women, there is some variation in them. In women, fat generally accumulates around the hips and in the thighs. In men, this accumulation is mostly in the abdominal area. But in the course of time, in chronic cases of obesity this accumulation of fat and muscle is not just localized, but covers the whole body.

Causes of Obesity

Though it is difficult to pinpoint the exact cause of obesity, it can be fairly stated that it is a result of overeating. Although other factors may also be involved, it is certain that, without excessive eating, generally there will not be obesity.

In treating obese patients at the Indian Institute of Yoga, Patna, and also at the Yoga Institute of Washington, D.C., I have found that all obese people develop certain common habits, make some common errors, and they all have the following common characteristics:[1]

   (i) They are addicted to overeating,
   (ii) They eat most of the time,
   (iii) All of them, without exception, eat fast without chewing food properly,
   (iv) They retire soon after dinner,

---

[1]The author founded the Yoga Institute of Washington in 1964 and taught yoga to more than 8,000 men and women until 1968. He had the opportunity to treat about 200 cases of obesity during his five years of yoga teaching.

The Indian Institute of Yoga, Patna, was founded in 1969 by the author and here also he has treated more than a hundred cases of obesity. The above observations are based on the findings of treating these persons.

(v) They either purposely avoid or do not have time to do physical labor and exercises.

We can say that obesity is the result of modern civilization. All classes of people in the developed nations and people of the upper classes in the developing nations are now getting more and better food and in many varieties than was possible years ago. Moreover, scientific developments and modern facilities have made the lives of the upper strata of society so comfortable that they hardly have any need to do physical labor for a living. In the absence of any physical work, on the one hand, and the daily intake of highly rich food, on the other, one is bound to add extra weight.

To have a clear picture of the life style of a modern man of a well-developed society, let me sketch briefly how he passes his day. A typical man's routine is like this: He gets up in the morning, shaves, washes, dresses, has a sumptuous breakfast, comes down in an elevator, gets into his car, rides to his office building, takes the elevator up, sits in his chair for office work, goes down in an elevator to a restaurant in the same building, has delicacies for lunch, comes back to his office, and sits there again until closing time, when he takes his car and returns home. At home during the evening, he watches television while drinking beer or some other drinks. Then he has a dinner of the choicest food and plenty of drinks. Without waiting for even an hour, he retires to bed and goes to sleep. He repeats the same routine the next day, the day after that, and so on.

As can be seen from the above pattern, the individual did not have to move around nor do any physical labor. On the other hand, he kept feeding himself the fatty, nourishing, and high-caloried food day and night. Therefore, the body gets more food than it needs for its balanced growth and upkeep. As a result, overweight develops and, in most cases, takes the form of obesity. When the individual passes his days as described above, he gets so used to his routine that he feels helpless and a victim of his own luxuries and comforts. Many become addicted to certain types of food and habits, and they need treatment to restore their normal health as any other patient of a chronic disease would need.

Another disheartening problem related to obesity is that the individual develops a feeling of inferiority. He does not like to meet his friends and social groups. He begins to isolate himself and lives a secluded life. In isolation or in the company of his own type, he prefers to eat something most of the time and develops certain bad habits such as drinking alcohol, using intoxicating drugs, and adopting other harmful ways of living. The individual so isolated develops various mental disorders such as nervousness, tension, anxiety, fear, or lack of confidence. Thus, he entraps himself in a sort of a vicious circle. When he is nervous and anxious, he eats to pacify himself. And eating ultimately brings him back to the same mental condition he was already suffering from. Finally, he develops many undesirable living habits and it becomes difficult to restore him to normal health.

Yoga Method of Correcting Obesity

The yoga method of correcting obesity primarily involves doing two things: (i) eating a balanced and proper diet, and (ii) practicing a few selected *asanas*. Before describing both these aspects, a few pertinent observations need to be made.

In treating obese persons at the Indian Institute of Yoga, Patna, and at the Yoga Institute of Washington, D.C., I have found that, according to our process, the average rate of weight reduction is 1 to 1½ pounds per week. An obese person loses about 4 to 6 pounds per month. Depending upon his total extra weight, the correction period for an obese person lasts for some months. For example, if a person carries 42 pounds of extra weight, the period for reducing this weight may be seven to ten months.

The biggest advantage of this yogic system of treatment is that the individual does not have to fast and he does not feel any weakness because the reduction in weight is gradual. Due to this gradual reduction, there is no sagging of the facial tissues or of the body's skin and muscles. In this process, weight reduction and body conditioning occur simultaneously. As a result, by the time the obese person has been restored to his normal weight, his body becomes proportionate.

It might be argued that the yogic system takes too long to reduce this excessive weight, whereas several manufacturers and advertisers of weight-reducing gadgets, food packages, pills, and drugs claim to reduce weight in a matter of days and weeks. Such advertisements probably attract millions of people by these claims. But these "gimmicks" do not bring any lasting results and may cause various ailments, disorders, and even serious physical-mental harm to the users. I have been shocked to see several young girls and boys in the United States and India ruin their health, beauty, and mental balance by using these "gimmicks" and "quickies."

The yoga method, though time consuming, is preferable and desirable for several reasons. It reduces weight permanently without causing any ill effects to health, beauty, and the physical-mental condition. It does not cost a penny to correct the disorder. There is no disturbance to normal life, nor is there any possibility of regaining the same weight even if yoga practice is discontinued and only the method of eating is maintained.

It is advised that, once the weight has been reduced to normal, the individual keep practicing yoga even for ten to fifteen minutes per day. If yoga practice is stopped, the individual should continue to follow the yogic principles and method of eating. By taking a proper and balanced diet, the normal weight will always remain the same. Overweight and obese persons are advised to eat according the diet chart given here.

Breakfast (6 to 9 A.M.)

   (i) Fruit juice or vegetable juice (with a little lemon juice   — ½ glass

   (ii) Fresh fruits (any kind)   — as desired

(iii) Sprouted chick-peas	— ½ cup
or	
Raw nuts (a mixture of unroasted cashews, almonds, pecans, walnuts, and pistachios)	— one handful
(iv) Wheat bread (without butter)	— one slice
or	
Wheat germ with skim milk	— one cup
(v) Egg (boiled or poached)	— one, if desired
(vi) Herb tea or decaffeinated coffee with milk and honey, or plain	— one cup, if desired

Lunch and Dinner (12 noon to 2 P.M. and 6 to 8 P.M.)

(i) Salad (a mixture of tomato, cucumber, radish, carrot, lettuce, beets, watercress, celery and sprouts) with salt, pepper, and lemon juice or with salad dressing, or plain	— one medium bowl
(ii) Soup (any kind)	— one cup
(iii) Whole wheat bread or rice	— as desired
(iv) Fresh green vegetables (boiled or stewed)	— as desired
(v) Leafy vegetables (any kind)	— as desired
(vi) Fish, liver, or seafood (for non-vegetarians)	— if desired, on alternate days
(vii) Non-fat yogurt	— one cup, if desired

Afternoon Refreshment (3 to 5 P.M.)

| *(i)* Fresh fruits (any kind) | — as desired |

(ii)	Green peas (roasted, steamed, or broiled)	— one cup
	or	
	Crackers	— one or two
(iii)	Herb tea or decaffeinated coffee with skim milk and without sugar	— one cup, if desired

The above-mentioned diet chart provides only an outline of items to be taken for breakfast, lunch, afternoon refreshment, and dinner. It does not explain the methods, principles, and essential requirements. Without observing these vitally important aspects, just eating according to the diet chart would not produce satisfactory results. The chart is meaningful and important only when the following principles, methods, and requirements are observed sincerely.

Principles and Requirements of Eating:

(i) The first and most important principle is to eat slowly after chewing and crushing the food thoroughly.

(ii) The second vitally important principle is to finish eating (especially dinner) at least two hours before sleeping at night.

(iii) The third and most important principle is: *Never eat more than eighty-five percent of your capacity at any time. Always eat a little less than you need.*

(iv) Avoid drinking water while eating. Drink water half an hour after eating. Take ten to fifteen glasses of fresh water in twenty-four hours.

(v) Do not eat fatty, fried, and highly seasoned food. Avoid hot spices, pickles, chutney, and sweets. Prepare your food with the least amount of spices for flavor.

(vi) Eat only four times in twenty-four hours: breakfast in the morning, lunch at noon, some light refreshment in the afternoon, and dinner at night. Avoid eating anything in between.

By following the principles and methods of eating described above and by practicing the yoga *asanas* mentioned below, you can be sure of losing a minimum of 6 pounds of weight every month.

Selected Yoga Asanas:

The overweight and the obese must practice yoga on a selected basis. It would not be possible for them to perform all types of *asanas* at the initial stage, nor is it necessary to do some of the difficult ones for the desired result. There are several *asanas* which are simple and easy to do, and have a remarkable effect on weight reduction and body conditioning. Therefore, practitioners are advised to begin their practice according to the selection of *asanas* given below.

Note: You should not try to do too many *asanas* in the beginning. Proceed gradually but regularly. Start with the *asanas* recommended for the first week and then add the *asanas* for the second, third, and other weeks. This way, your progress would be gradual, steady, and without any strain and exhaustion. The results will begin to show right from the first week, even though you would be practicing only a few yoga *asanas*. With these clarifications, let me recommend what you need to practice during the first week and afterwards.

First Week of Yoga Practice

During the first week, start with the following *asanas:*
   1. *Ekpada Utthan asana:* as described in Chapter 4. Make a total of eight rounds—four rounds with each leg alternately.
   2. *Uttanapada asana:* as described in Chapter 2. Make a total of only four rounds daily; never do more than six rounds in a day.

Rest: After practicing the above *asanas*, rest in *Shava asana* for five minutes. See Chapter 2 for the way to practice *Shava asana*.

Second Week of Yoga Practice

Keep practicing both the *asanas* of the first week and add the following:

> 3. *Bhujanga asana:* as described in Chapter 2. Practice four rounds daily.
> 4. *Shalabha asana:* as described in Chapter 2. Practice four rounds daily.

After performing all four *asanas*, rest in *Shava asana* for five minutes.

Third Week of Yoga Practice

Keep practicing all four *asanas* of the preceding weeks and add the following ones at the start of the third week:

> 5. *Santulan asana:* as described in Chapter 5. Make a total of six rounds with each side, alternately.
> 6. *Pawana Mukta asana:* as described in Chapter 2. Make a total of six rounds daily—do three rounds with each side, alternately.

After practicing all six *asanas*, rest in *Shava asana* for seven minutes.

Fourth Week of Yoga Practice

Keep practicing all six *asanas* of the preceding weeks and add the following ones at the beginning of the fourth week:

> 7. *Surya Namaskar asana:* as described in Chapter 3. Make four rounds daily.
> 8. *Dhanur asana:* as described in Chapter 3. Make four rounds daily.

After practicing all eight *asanas*, rest in *Shava asana* for ten minutes.

Fifth Week of Yoga Practice

Keep practicing all eight *asanas* of the preceding weeks and add the following ones at the beginning of the fifth week:

9. *Ardha Vakra asana:* as described in Chapter 3. Make only four rounds daily—two rounds with each side.
10. *Pashchimottan asana:* as described in Chapter 2. Make only four rounds daily.

After practicing all the *asanas,* rest for ten minutes in *Shava asana.*

Sixth Week and Afterwards

Add the following *asanas* during the sixth week and in your later practice:

11. *Supta Vajra asana:* as described in Chapter 3. Make only four rounds daily.
12. *Matsyendra asana:* as described in Chapter 3. Make only four rounds daily—two rounds with each side.
13. *Manduka asana:* as described below.

MANDUKA ASANA
(FROG POSE)

Position of Readiness: To do this *asana,* you need a padded floor. Therefore, put a blanket or folded cloth on the floor. Sit on your folded legs, as shown in Figure 15. You should be in the same position as you have to be in the sitting position for making *Supta Vajra asana.* Sit in this position and breathe normally. This is the position of readiness.

Steps of Actual Practice: (i) By placing more body weight on the right foot, lessen the weight on the left foot. This will make it possible for you to put the left foot under the left side of the hip.

(ii) Then, by putting the body's weight on the left side, bring the right foot under the right hip. Now you are sitting on the floor and your left foot is folded on the left side and the right foot is folded on the right side. Keep the palms on the floor to support the body. If this is painful, do not proceed further;

practice only this for some time. When you have no difficulty in reaching this stage, proceed with the following steps:

(iii) While keeping the hands on the floor on both sides and partially supporting the body weight, separate the knees gradually. Move the left knee further to the left and the right knee to the right. Try to separate them as much as you can comfortably.

(iv) When the knees have been separated to a feasible point, stay there and do the following: Bring the palms on the knees on their respective sides. Keep the body straight and look in front. Breathe normally. Remain in this position for eight to twelve seconds. You should be in the position shown in Figure 43.

(v) After staying in that position for the desired time, return to the sitting position by the following method: Put your palms on the floor and then kneel. Now bring forward any foot in front first by sliding it under the hip. Now bring the other leg in front. Then sit comfortably and relax. After resting for six to eight seconds, repeat this *asana* a few times more by following the same process.

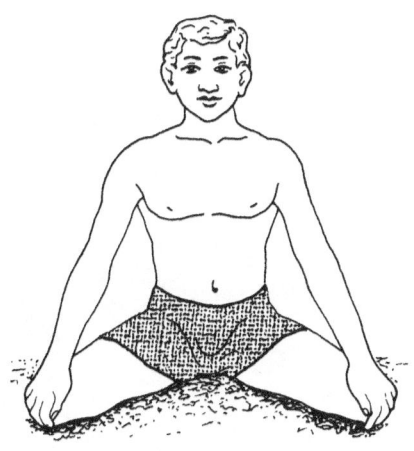

Figure 43. Manduka Asana

Daily Practice: Twice daily during the first week. Gradually develop the practice to a maximum of four times daily.

Benefits: This is a very effective *asana* for reducing the weight of the thighs, hips, and abdominal areas. For both men and women, it conditions the muscles and nerves of the lower areas of the body.

This *asana* has several other benefits. It activates all the joints of the lower body, enhances sexual potency, corrects disorders of the reproductive system, cures piles, and strengthens the digestive system. With a little effort, this *asana* can be practiced by anyone.

CHAPTER 7

Mental Problems

The mind loses its equilibrium when any external or internal problem strains it greatly. Consequently, its functioning is disturbed and its harmony begins to diminish, slowly or rapidly, depending upon the individual's state of mental health. The person so affected for a long time becomes mentally ill, with an intensity proportionate to the degree of the harmony lost. Thus, the individual's thoughts, actions, manner, behavior, and outlook become imbalanced, resulting in various forms and shapes of abnormal expressions. This problem can affect people of any age, sex, socioeconomic background, and country. Here we are faced then with two problems: (i) how to correct and cure the cases of mental sickness, and (ii) how can one maintain sound mental health. The answer to both problems is found in the yoga system.

Causes of Mental Problems

In order to make the methodological processes of yoga comprehensible, a brief discussion about the causes of mental problems is essential. All troubles which affect the mind spring from three basic sources: (i) *Nature*, (ii) *Society*, and (iii) *Self*. In other words, problems which strain and cause a mental imbalance in an individual are either nature-oriented, society-oriented, or self-oriented and have been termed as *Daivik*, *Bhautik*, and *Atmik* by Kapil in his Samkhya philosophy.

The problems arising from nature could be in the form of some natural calamity, danger from certain creatures, and peculiar natural phenomena. Societal problems, likewise, could be religious, ethnic, racial, economic, or political; or they might also involve such problems as adjusting to certain customs, manners, and the ways of life of a particular community. Similarly, there could be countless problems of an individual's own creation which are caused by certain beliefs, faith, notions, habits, manners, and also because of some inner feelings such as hatred, jealousy, revenge, love, romance, likes, and dislikes.

People of every society—be it industrial, agrarian, tribal, or primitive—have been faced with various problems caused by these three sources, more or less in the same way that we have to face them today. Though the nature, forms, and shapes of human problems have changed because of changes in social conditions, they basically remain the same. Seen in this context, it would be interesting to know what the early thinkers of yoga have thought about these problems and what solutions they have provided.

Among the forefathers whose contribution became the foundation of the Yoga System is that of Kapil. Therefore, let us see what Kapil had to say about this problem.

The contribution of Kapil (700 B.C.) is called Samkhya philosophy.[1] According to Kapil, the answer to all human problems is in *samyak jnana* (proper knowledge). In the absence of *samyak jnana*, unfamiliar and peculiar events cause *dukha* (sorrow). When the individual develops and acquires

---

[1]The most authentic book available on Samkhya philosophy is by Ishwar Krishna, *Samkhya Karika* (Delhi: Motilal Banarsi Das). 1966.

proper knowledge about *Purusha* (Self) and *Prakriti* (Nature), then such events caused by any of the three mentioned sources do not cause *dukha*. This implies acquiring a scientific knowledge of *rajas, tamas,* and *sattva gunas,* and all the *tattvas* (elements) of *Prakriti,* together with a knowledge of the composition, function, and co-relationship of the sense and action organs, mind, intelligence, and the totality of the *Purusha* (Self). When the individual becomes so knowledgeable, he attains the power to overcome pain; maintains mental equilibrium; and obtains pleasure, happiness, and excellence in life.

But this Samkhya philosophy did not provide the method and process of obtaining the goal. A more comprehensive system was needed to help the individual to adopt and achieve what had been so rightly stated by Kapil. This system was provided by Patanjali in his *Yoga Sutra*.

Patanjali's Yoga Sutra

The *Yoga Sutra* of Patanjali (300 B.C.) is a treatise on the methodology of obtaining the goal laid down by Kapil and adds something more. Whereas Kapil emphasized acquiring *jnana,* which involves only the mind, Patanjali's system of yoga involves both mind and body. In this respect, the *Purusha* of Patanjali must do two things simultaneously: he must acquire *samyak jnana* and he must perform yoga practices to achieve excellence of both body and mind. By combining *jnana* and practices, the individual would attain not only excellent health but would also be able to maintain harmony between the mind and the body. Thus, we find that Patanjali's yoga provides a better and more thorough answer to our mental health problems than that provided by Kapil.

Since Patanjali's system involves both knowing and doing, his method includes all those steps which are essential for obtaining the desired goal on both levels—physical and mental. These steps are eight in number. They are mentioned below, together with their basic meanings and implications:

Yama (control and discipline), *Niyama* (rules, methods, and principles), *Asanas* (making body postures), *Pranayamas* (*kriyas* with air), *Pratyahara* (avoidance of undesirables in taking actions; that is, knowing the proper action), *Dharana* (concentration), *Dhyana* (meditation), and *Samadhi* (contemplation).

Since these eight steps of Patanjali were not very comprehensively discussed in his *Yoga Sutra,* further works were necessary to cover them properly. To make it more convenient for practitioners, these steps were later grouped, according to their nature and substance, under different yogas. The yogas which cover all these steps are the following four:

JNANA YOGA covers *Yama* and *Niyama* and is the science of acquiring proper knowledge.

HATHA YOGA covers *Asanas* and *Pranayamas* and is the science of physical excellence.

KARMA YOGA covers *Pratyahara* and is the science of action.

RAJA YOGA covers *Dharana, Dhyana,* and *Samadhi* and is the science of concentration and meditation.

Applied Yoga

It must be clearly stated here that not all types of mental cases can be helped through yoga. This limitation becomes imperative because it is assumed that those going to practice yoga have the mental capability to understand its basic principles, methods, and thoughts, and are physically able to perform even the simplest practices. Unless these basic requirements about the physical and mental status are fulfilled, it would be difficult for persons concerned to properly use yoga. With this understanding, the process of treatment and steps are described here. These recommendations are based on our experiences in correcting and curing various cases of mental illness at the Indian Institute of Yoga, Patna.

Jnana and Karma Yogas: Persons suffering from mental disorders are advised to know the basic tenets of Jnana Yoga and Karma Yoga. Both these yogas relate to the essentials of *samyak jnana* (acquiring proper knowledge) and of *satkarvavad* (science of action). These yogas involve knowing certain basic concepts, theories, principles, and thoughts concerning the **Self, Society,** and **Nature.** A knowledge of these would equip the individual to understand the causes and effects of a given situation and would make him know how to act properly to obtain a satisfactory result. This being the importance of these two yogas,[2] the individual should know them along with the practices of Hatha Yoga.

Guidelines: To achieve the fullest benefit of yoga, it is important that practitioners have a proper understanding of the "Essentials of Yoga Practice." These essentials have been briefly described in Chapter 1. People with mental problems are advised to read the first chapter with special attention to (a) therapeutic yoga, (b) essentials of yoga practice, (c) proper diet, and (d) bathing and cleaning. A proper understanding of these points and their adoption would provide a very satisfactory result to practitioners.

With the knowledge of the first chapter, they should begin practicing Hatha Yoga according to the stages and steps outlined below:

Hatha Yoga: Hatha Yoga is comprised of *pranayamas, asanas, bandhas,* and *mudras.* People with mental problems are advised to practice only some of the selected items in the initial stage. When their normal mental condition is restored, they could try other items of Hatha Yoga according to their own preference. With this understanding they are recommended to begin their practice on the following basis:

---

[2]For a proper understanding of these yogas, read Swami Vivekananda, *The Yoga and Other Works* (New York: Ramakrishna-Vivekananda Centre, 1955). Both *Jnana Yoga* and *Karma Yoga* are included in this edition. These books are available in Hindi and other languages in India and have been published by the Ramakrishna Mission.

First Week of Yoga Practice

They should begin with *Ujjayee Pranayama* in the Lying Position. It is easy and any person can do it. The method of practicing *Ujjayee* in the Lying Position is fully described in Chapter 4. Only five rounds of it should be done daily.

After making five rounds of *Ujjayee*, they should practice *Surya Namaskar asana* and *Uttanapada asana*. Four rounds of each of the above two *asanas* would be sufficient. Do not do more than four rounds of each. Follow the method of doing *Surya Namaskar* given in Chapter 3 and that of *Uttanapada* as described in Chapter 2.

When all of these three items have been practiced, the practitioner should rest either in *Shava asana* or by just lying on the back and breathing normally. After doing all three items, one should rest for five minutes.

Second and Third Week of Yoga Practice

During the second week, the following *asanas* should be added:

Pashchimottan asana: as described in Chapter 2.
Bhujanga asana: as described in Chapter 2.
Trikona asana: as described in Chapter 5.

After practicing all of the *asanas* and the *pranayama* mentioned above, the practitioner should now rest in *Shava asana* (as described in Chapter 2) for ten to fifteen minutes.

Fourth Week Onward Yoga Practice

During the fourth week, practitioners should gradually add either all the *asanas* given below or choose and practice only those which they can perform comfortably:

Sarvanga asana: as described in Chapter 4.
Matsya asana: as described in Chapter 4.

Dhanur asana: as described in Chapter 3.
Hala asana: as described below.

HALA ASANA
(PLOUGH POSE)

This *asana* is one of the best in the Hatha Yoga system. Because of some unique qualities and excellent benefits, it occupies a very prominent place in the list of *asanas*.

This *asana* can be performed in two ways. Though one form is easier than the other, both have almost the same effects and rewards. Since it is a valuable *asana*, the methodology of both forms is described and explained separately. Let me present the easier one first.

Form 1

Position of Readiness: Lie flat on your back. Stretch out the whole body, keeping it very straight. Bring the heels and toes together. Place the palms on the floor quite close to the body on both sides. Straighten your neck and head. You should be in the same readiness position as for *Uttanapada asana*.

Actual Performance: First stretch out the legs and tense them. Also stretch the toes and point them opposite to the direction of the head. Now inhale and simultaneously raise both legs

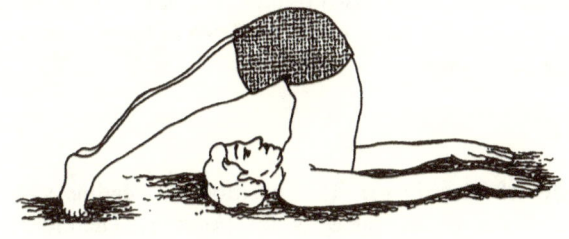

Figure 44. Hala Asana (Easy Pose)

upward until they are vertical. Synchronize inhaling and lifting the legs. Keep both palms on the floor.

Second, when you have reached the vertical point, start exhaling and simultaneously start lowering the legs back over the head. Try to touch the floor behind the head as far as the toes can possibly reach. Go back only as far as is possible for you. Stay at the point where you can and stabilize yourself there. After the exhaling is over, breathe normally until the whole posture is completed. You should now be as shown in Figure 44. Remain in this position for about eight to ten seconds. You are now in the Plough Pose.

Note: As long as you are in this second phase, keep the legs quite taut and do not bend them at the knees. Keep the toes stretched and pointing to or touching the ground. Keep both palms on the floor and the arms and hands straight and quite firm.

Third, after remaining in the second phase for about ten seconds, start returning the back to the floor. Control this returning phase. Let the back roll down to the floor, inch by inch. It is very important that you return gradually, slowly, and smoothly. Keep the legs and toes quite tensed during the returning phase; they should be very stiff. When the heels touch the ground, relax the whole body. You have completed one round of the Plough Pose. Now relax for six to eight seconds. Then try some more rounds in the same manner as the first one.

Limitation: Begin with two rounds. Increase it to a maximum of four rounds. A regular practice of two to three rounds should be quite satisfactory.

Form 2

Position of Readiness: The position of readiness for this Second Form is the same as for Form 1. Therefore, make yourself ready according to the directions given there.

Actual Performance: First inhale and raise both arms up parallel, like two sticks. Bring the arms back over the head and place the back of the hands on the floor, parallel to each other. You should synchronize your inhaling and lifting the arms so that by the time your hands have touched the floor you are still inhaling. When the hands touch the floor, exhale.

Second, soon after this exhaling is over, start inhaling and, at the same time, start lifting both legs up to a vertical position.

When the legs are vertical, start exhaling and, at the same time, start lowering the legs back over your head towards the floor and above the fingers. Now put your toes on the floor. If you cannot touch the floor with the toes, go only as far down as is possible for you. After this last exhaling is over, keep breathing normally; do not hold the breath. Stabilize yourself in a position which is comfortable.

At this point, pay attention to the following things: Your legs should remain as stiff as sticks. The toes should be stretched out on or near the floor. Do not slacken or bend the knees. Try to keep the arms, hands, and palms parallel to one another. When these requirements are fulfilled, you are in a perfect Plough Posture as shown in Figure 45. Remain in this phase for about ten seconds.

Third, after being in the Plough Pose for about ten seconds, return gradually and in a controlled way according to the following method. This returning process is as important as performing the posture itself. Therefore, concentrate on a

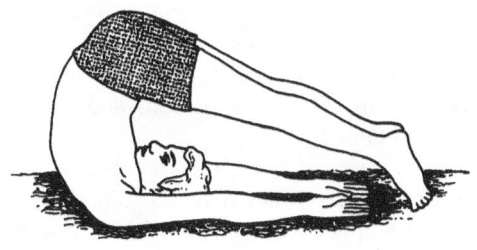

Figure 45. Hala Asana

smooth, slow, and controlled return. Let the shoulders roll back first, then the hips, and, lastly, the thighs, legs, and heels, in that order. Try to roll back inch by inch.

While returning, keep the hands on the floor where they are. Withdraw only the legs. Roll back the whole body and let the heels fall on the floor. When the heels have touched the floor, lift both hands up and return them, like two parallel sticks, to the floor. Now place the palms on the floor. You have completed one round of the best form of the Plough Posture. Now relax. Let the whole body be loose. Relax for about six to eight seconds. Then make a few more rounds in the same manner as the first one.

Limitation: Make one round on the first day. Gradually go to four rounds in a few days. Four rounds are the maximum.

Benefits: The Plough Posture has some special values. According to Tantra Yoga, it is the unique *asana* for gaining sexual powers. It invigorates, energizes, and nourishes all the sexual glands and increases their power, strength, and vitality. Further, it has curative and corrective values for any weakened condition of the sex glands. Because of these values, it has a curative effect on impotency, frigidity, and lack of sexual power.

There are several other excellent benefits of this *asana*. It exercises every inch of the backbone. The whole spinal cord is normalized and soothed. Thus, as far as the flexibility of the spine is concerned, it surpasses all other *asanas* in its effects.

The Plough Posture is excellent for reducing weight. It removes excess weight without weakening the body. It makes the body proportionate by reducing the waistline, by toning up the digestive system, by taking off fat, and by activating the whole nervous system.

It also has a very good effect on the facial area. Since there is an increase in the circulation of the blood which becomes centralized in the upper regions, the Plough Posture nourishes the whole area and thereby increases and restores the youthful look of the face.

Note: After doing the above-mentioned *asanas*, the practitioner should rest for ten to fifteen minutes in *Shava asana*. When the practice of *pranayama* and *asanas* has been regularized for about a month, the practice of concentration, as described below, should be added.

CONCENTRATION

Concentration is the primary step of Raja Yoga. Its next advanced stage is meditation. Before describing how to practice concentration, let me explain briefly what it is and what it does.[3]

Concentration means one pointedness of the mind according to the will of the individual. By acquiring this power, the individual becomes the master of his own mind and controls its fluctuations. His mind is not allowed the freedom to wander and attach itself to countless issues, events, thoughts, and objects. In concentration, the involvement of the mind becomes selective and for some desirable purpose; meaningless and worthless attachment is eliminated. When this power of concentration is achieved through proper training, it has a great curative effect on mental sickness. This curative effect can be understood better when the nature of the mind and also the mind-body relationship are explained.

The mind, by its nature, always tries to associate itself with many issues, events, objects, or thoughts. Its involvement is with only one thing at a time, and this time may be short or long. To what it will attach itself is unpredictable.

This associative nature of the mind creates one specific condition in the body which must be understood. The nature of the objects, issues, or events to which the mind attaches itself generates a similar reaction in the body. In other words, the nature of reaction is the same as is the nature of the object of involvement. Accordingly, when the mind attaches to some-

---

[3]For more on concentration, see Dr. Phulgenda Sinha. *Yoga: Meaning, Values and Practice* (Bombay: Jaico Publishing House, 1972), pp. 15-32.

thing which, by its nature, could arouse anger in the individual, then it will generate in his body all those conditions and changes which anger arouses by its very nature. The uncalled-for attachment of the mind, by its nature, would arouse uncalled-for conditioning of his bodily system, resulting at times in tension, excitement, and temper; and, at others, into pleasure and thrill. It is strongly held in yoga that, unless the distraction of the mind is controlled and the mind's energy is properly channeled towards a desired purpose, nothing worthwhile can be accomplished by the individual. This ability to control the mind and to channel it in the chosen direction is achieved through the training in concentration. To practice concentration, you must make certain preparations as described below:

Arranging the Object: Place a vase with a flower in it on a piece of furniture low enough so that the top of the flower is at the level of your eyes when you are in the sitting position. The flower can be natural or artificial. There should be a distance of about five feet between the object and the practitioner. Also, there should be enough light on the object.

Method of Practicing Concentration: When the flower is arranged properly, be seated in an easy pose as shown in Figure 46. To make this easy pose, bend both legs at the knees and put the body's weight on the floor. Then place the left hand in the lap and the right hand on the palm of the left. This will make your right palm upwards on top of the left palm.

Then sit erect so that your head, neck, and spine are in one line. After the body has been straightened, do not tighten it. Rather, let the body be relaxed while keeping it firm and upright. Breathe normally. You are now in *Sukha asana* (Easy Pose) as shown in Figure 46 and ready to begin the practice of *dharana* (concentration), the first step in controlling the fluctuation of the mind. Follow the steps suggested below:

Look at the flower petals for about ten seconds. If you feel any pain in the eyes, look for a shorter time. Try not to blink

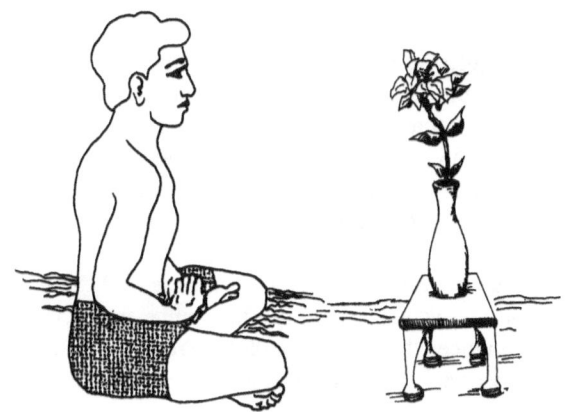

Figure 46. Practice of Concentration

the eyes. When you have looked at the flower for ten seconds, close your eyes gently and try to see the shape of the flower in your mind. Keep your eyes closed for about ten seconds while trying to recall the image and shape of the flower in your mind. After keeping the eyes closed for only ten seconds, open them and again look at the flower for ten seconds. Repeat this process of seeing, closing, and seeing; that is, seeing through the eyes, closing the eyes, and then seeing through the inner eye. Repeat this process only five times in one session during the first week. Gradually increase it up to ten and then up to fifteen times, which should remain the limit. Here, "time" means "round." Ten times would mean ten rounds. If you practice only ten rounds in one session, that is quite sufficient. But, *never* go beyond fifteen rounds in a single session.

When the practice is over, keep sitting still. Then loosen the body and sit in a relaxed way for two minutes. When you have done this, your practice in concentration is complete.

Some Suggestions: It is suggested that, after practicing with a single flower for about a month, you may add more flowers in the vase, although this addition is not necessary.

It is also suggested that, after two months of practicing with flowers, you could change the object. You could then practice with a photo, statue, or painting of your liking. The only consideration which you should have about the object is its size, color, and type. The object should be of medium size, of bright color, and be soothing and pleasing, but never thrilling.

Caution: Practitioners of concentration must read the following warnings and always keep them in mind while practicing. As in any other science, the rules of Raja Yoga should also be cautiously observed to avoid undesirable consequences. Thus, the following warnings:

The first warning is about the time limitation. The total time devoted to this practice of concentration should not exceed more than ten to fifteen minutes. Unless the teacher is personally guiding the procedure, practitioners should limit the whole period of concentration to only ten to fifteen minutes within a period of twenty-four hours.

The imposed limitation is necessary for some good reasons. One is that some practitioners might become fascinated by the peculiar images flashing before their inner eye during concentration. This fascination, unless checked, might mislead the practitioner into misusing his time. Second, if one keeps practicing for the sake of thrills and fascination, he is not only diverting himself from the desired goal, but is also risking some unknown consequences which might have ill effects on his actions, thoughts, performances, and behavior. A time limit, therefore, will always keep the practitioner safe from undesirable consequences.

Testing Concentration: You can test yourself to determine whether you have gained concentration or not. Use the following guidelines: While practicing, when you do not see anything through the inner eye, you have not gained concentration. While practicing, when you see some other object through your inner eye but not the one placed before your outer eyes, you are improving but still have not gained concentration. But when you see the shape of the actual object through the inner eye, even for a second, you have gained concentration. When the object remains before the inner eye, in any form and shape, for up to five seconds, you have gained good concentration. When you can hold the same shape or image for up to ten seconds, you have gained a very high level of concentration. And when you have gained concentration, your mental sickness or disorders are gone and you are fully restored to normal.

CHAPTER 8

Neck and Spinal Pain

Since both these ailments are related to the spine, they are covered together in this chapter.

NECK PAIN

In medical terminology, neck pain affecting the cervical spine is called Cervical Spondylosis. This pain can spread to both sides of the shoulders, the back of the neck, the collar-bone, and the shoulder joints. In some cases, the pain might be in both arms and also in their joints.

In the medical system of treatment, patients are given medicines, heat compresses, and a neck collar. Though these aids provide some relief, they do not guarantee a complete cure. Being uncertain of their medicinal effect, it is not uncommon for medical men to advise their patients to also do some physical exercises to relieve the pain. From our experience, we have found that such physical exercises are less effective when compared to yoga postures. This is evident from the fact that, while there is an uncertainty of cure through physical exercises and medicines, there is the certainty of complete cure through yoga without any medicines. Before describing the yogic method of treatment, let me explain briefly the causes and cure of this ailment.

Causes and Cure: The causes of neck pain can be several. It could be due to the regular use of a very high pillow under the head while sleeping. Another reason could be keeping the head bent in a particular position for a long time instead of keeping it erect. It could also be due to the rigidity of the muscles and nerves in the neck and shoulder areas which obstructs the proper circulation of blood.

The yogic method of treatment requires (i) eating a proper diet, (ii) correcting errors and faulty habits, and (iii) practicing some selected yoga *asanas*. The diet for those with neck pain is the same as recommended for arthritic patients in Chapter 5. To obtain the full benefits of yoga, patients are also advised to read Chapter 1 to understand the yogic method of treatment and the essential requirements of its practice.

The patient should use a thin pillow while sleeping and avoid excessive bending of the neck. The rigidity of the muscles and the defective blood circulation will be automatically corrected through yoga practice.

Yoga Practice: The following asanas are recommended: During the first week, practice only the *Vriksha asana, Trikona asana,* and *Bhujanga asana.* After completing these three *asanas, Shava asana* should be done for three minutes.

From the second week onwards, practice all the *asanas* in the order listed below. After performing these six *asanas*, do the *Shava asana* for five to seven minutes.

Asanas to cure neck pain:

> *Vriksha asana:* as described in Chapter 5.
> *Trikona asana:* as described in Chapter 5.
> *Bhujanga asana:* as described in Chapter 2.
> *Gomukha asana:* as described in Chapter 5.
> *Veera asana:* as described in Chapter 5.
> *Jalandhar bandha:* as described below.

JALANDHAR BANDHA

Position of Readiness: Sit on the floor either in *Padma asana* (Lotus Pose) as shown in Figure 1 or in *Sukha asana* as shown in Figure 2 in Chapter 2. Keep the spine, neck, and head absolutely erect and in one line. Look straight ahead at eye level. Place your wrists on their respective sides of the knees, as shown in Figure 47. Breathe normally. You are now ready to do the *Jalandhar bandha*. Follow the steps below:

Steps of Actual Practice: (i) Inhale slowly, taking in as much air as you comfortably can.

(ii) Hold the breath and bend your head downwards slowly so that the chin touches the chest. Do not strain yourself while bending your head. If the chin does not touch the chest, go down as low as you can and stay there.

(iii) After the chin has touched the chest or is close to it, raise both shoulders upwards a little. Keep your spine erect and your head and neck straight while you hold the breath.

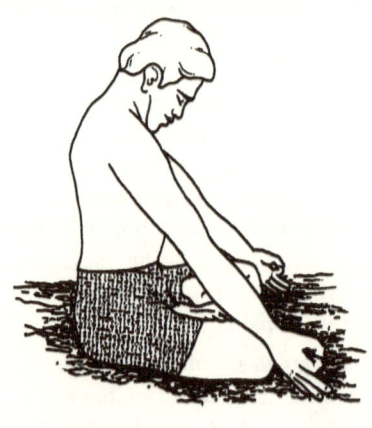

Figure 47. Jalandhar Bandha

(iv) Stay in this position for four to eight seconds while retaining your breath. This completes the *Jalandhar bandha*.

(v) Now raise your head gradually. As the chin leaves the chest, start exhaling slowly. When the head is straight and you have exhaled, rest for two normal breaths; i.e., breathe in and out without holding the air.

(vi) After resting for two breaths, repeat this *bandha* the same way as before.

Daily Practice: Four rounds daily. Start with three during the first week and then go up to four rounds from the second week onwards.

Benefits: This *bandha* cures disorders of the head, shoulders, and the cervical regions. It is also good for curing any disorder of the throat and face. People suffering from sinus and breathing problems will find this *bandha* very beneficial. It is easy to do and can be performed by anyone of any age.

SPINAL PAIN

Here, spinal pain refers to disorders and pains of the spine, particularly in the waist region. This pain, commonly called low backache, can spread to both sides of the waist and hips. When the pain is acute, the patient is almost made an invalid because any free physical movement is difficult. In acute conditions, the patient is bedridden.

Generally, people who are overweight develop spinal pain as they grow older. I have even found some young people suffering from this pain. Low backache might be tolerable in its initial stage and the individual might be able to bear it for some years. But prolonged pain of this type becomes chronic and gets aggravated in its later stages.

Causes and Cure: There are four main causes for this disorder: (i) faulty eating habits that result in overweight or underweight,

(ii) exposure to the cold, (iii) physical straining of the spine, and (iv) a bad sitting posture for a considerable length of time.

It has been found that a large number of people who suffer from spinal pain habitually drink water or tea, or both, after getting up in the morning. This regular drinking of water and tea upon arising leads to forced elimination of the bowels, which in turn weakens the digestive system. An empty stomach affects the condition of the spine, especially when the individual bathes or is exposed to the cold. The area near the waist becomes strained due to exposure and the person develops spinal pain. Excessive weight might be another reason for straining the spine. Pain could also be caused by some sudden physical strain or to habitually defective ways of sitting.

We have found that spinal pain is fully and permanently cured by yogic methods. It is only the restoration and correction period which varies. If the pain has been present for one year, it may take two months or more to cure it fully. If the pain has been there for less than a year, restoration could be complete within four to five weeks.

The yogic method of treatment involves eating a correct diet, sleeping on not too soft a bed, and practicing some selected *asanas*. The diet for patients with spinal pain is the same as recommended for arthritic patients in Chapter 5. A special advice is to stop taking tea or water upon arising in the morning. It would be better if tea and coffee were stopped completely for two months. Patients should not eat bananas and yogurt, and they should avoid eating fatty, spicy, and fried foods. For a better understanding of a correct diet, they are advised to read Chapter 1.

After making these clarifications and recommendations, let me describe the *asanas* to be practiced for curing spinal pain. Begin your yoga practice as described below:

Yoga Asanas for the First Week: During the first week, practice the following *asanas:*

    (i)   *Pawana Mukta asana:* (in the lying position) as described in Chapter 2.

(ii) *Bhujanga asana:* as described in Chapter 2.
(iii) *Shalabha asana:* (with one leg at a time) as described in Chapter 2.
(iv) *Uttanapada asana:* (with one leg at a time) as described in Chapter 2.
(v) *Shava asana:* for three minutes, as described in Chapter 2.

Second Week and Afterwards: From the second week onwards, the order of yoga practice should be:

(i) *Pawana Mukta asana:* in the lying position.
(ii) *Bhujanga asana:* moderately and without any strain.
(iii) *Shalabha asana:* with one leg at a time.
(iv) *Uttanapada asana:* with one leg at a time.
(v) *Ekpada Utthan asana:* as described in Chapter 4.
(vi) *Rechaka-Puraka Pranayama:* as described in Chapter 2.
(vii) *Shava asana:* for five to seven minutes.

By following the recommendation on diet and on other aspects, and by the daily practice of the yoga *asanas* listed above, you will be completely cured of all the disorders and pains in the neck and in the spinal regions without any medicinal aid.

CHAPTER 9

Sinus and Headache

Both these disorders are related to the head. Whereas sinus problems mainly affect the respiratory system and the nasal passages, headaches might occur in different parts of the head. Both ailments are discussed in this chapter.

SINUS (Sinusitis)

Sinusitis is a very common disorder—millions all over the world suffer from this very painful problem. Its symptoms vary from case to case. There is excessive or constant sneezing, drainage from the nose, blockage of one or both nostrils, heaviness of the head, or headache. In some cases, one or more of these symptoms may be present. It makes the life of the patient miserable because of constant sneezing, and, at times, complete congestion. Breathing is also very difficult. Due to the regular blocking of the nose, the voice is also affected. Chronic sinusitis affects the voice badly.

In the medical system of treatment, sinus problems are regarded as a result of allergies. Doctors try to find out the particular allergents to which the patient is sensitive. Medicines and injections are given in accordance with the identified allergent to develop a resistance in the patients. It is a very lengthy process and even then there is no certainty of curing the disorder.

I have found that though medicinal aids give momentary relief, they do not provide any permanent cure. It is a common practice to advise the patients to avoid using or contacting certain widely known allergents such as particular spices, flowers, perfumes, smoke, certain plants and animals, and countless other things. The yogic system of treatment is very different from the medical system. Let me describe what we consider the causes and cure of this trouble.

Causes and Cure: From my experience in treating patients with sinus trouble at the Yoga Institute of Washington, D.C., and at the Indian Institute of Yoga, Patna, I have found that a faulty diet is the primary cause of sinus trouble. When an individual takes certain types of foods or drinks regularly, in due time they greatly affect the whole bodily system.

Those who keep taking these foods or drinks constantly develop a sensitivity in their bodies. As a result, some become more sensitive to certain types of allergents, which ultimately results in sinusitis. Let me elaborate this point.

Many people are in the habit of drinking water upon arising in the morning; some take water first, then tea or coffee; some only take coffee or tea. Drinking tea or water on an empty stomach makes the bowel movement easy; but it has been found that such people develop a greater sensitivity to various things they use daily and also to the environment they live in. Then, there are people who eat fried food most of the time. This also affects the digestive system in due time and creates greater sensitivity. Some habitually drink milk either before going to sleep at night or during the day. The regular use of milk in heavy doses also causes sensitivity. When a person takes the above-mentioned items regularly, sensitivity increases and he or she is affected by various types of allergents which first turn into allergy and later on take the form of sinusitis.

In the yogic system of treatment, the main emphasis is on correcting the faulty diet. Patients are advised to eat a balanced diet and to avoid certain items which are considered undesirable, unnecessary, and unhealthy. They are recommended to eat only those foods which are considered good and healthy. The sinus patient should avoid the following: (i) tea or water after getting up in the morning; (ii) milk at any time, though certain milk preparations can be taken at times; (iii) perfumes and hair oils with a strong smell; (iv) fried foods; (v) eating butter regularly; and (vi) using sharp or hot spices.

The diet chart for patients with sinus trouble is the same as recommended for patients with abdominal disorders in Chapter 2, and they are advised to follow it.

By eating the suggested diet, and by following the *pranayamas* recommended below, patients should be cured of sinus trouble within two to three weeks.

Yoga Practice: Practice the following *pranayamas* for curing the sinus disorder:

> *(i) Rechaka-Puraka pranayama:* as described in Chapter 2; see Figures 1 and 2.
>
> (ii) *Bhastrika pranayama:* as described below.
>
> (iii) *Shava asana:* for five minutes, as described in Chapter 2.

BHASTRIKA PRANAYAMA

The ideal time for practicing the *Bhastrika pranayama* is in the morning before breakfast. It is important to practice it when the stomach is empty. Those who would like to do it in the evening or at some other time must allow three or four hours to elapse after eating.

Position of Readiness: Be seated on some padded surface

either in the Lotus Pose or in *Sukha asana* as shown in Figures 1 and 2. Keep your head and spine erect. Keep your hands on your knees as shown in Figure 48. Look directly in front and breathe normally. Keep the mouth closed. This is the position of readiness for *Bhastrika pranayama*.

Steps of Actual Practice: In this *pranayama*, the stomach is pulled in and then brought forward in a quick succession with every exhalation and inhalation. While exhaling, the stomach is pulled inside and while inhaling, the stomach is pushed forward. It is done like the bellows of the blacksmith. To make the *Bhastrika pranayama*, follow the steps described below:

(i) During the first phase, start gradually and slowly to exhale the air through both nostrils and, at the same time, start to pull the stomach inside. After you have exhaled the air fully, begin inhaling and, at the same time, start pushing the stomach forward. One exhalation and one inhalation comprise one unit of *Bhastrika pranayama*.

Note: Do not pull the stomach upward or downward during this *pranayama*.

(ii) After doing three or four units slowly and gradually,

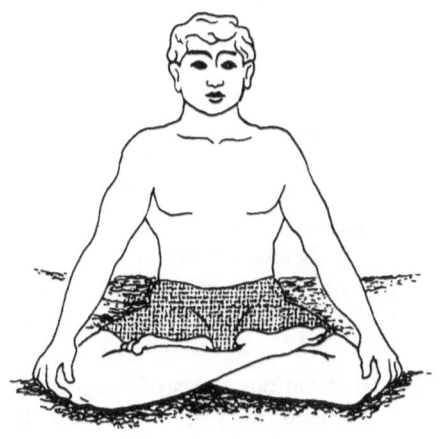

Figure 48.   Bhastrika Pranayama

begin to breathe fast in quick successions. Make five to six inhalations and exhalations, one after another, rapidly during this second phase.

(iii) Gradually slow down your speed. Breathe three to four times slowly in this last phase. Then rest for three to four normal breaths. Resting should take about twenty seconds. While resting, remain seated easily by relaxing the body either in the same position or by sitting as comfortably as you like.

(iv) After resting for the desired period, repeat the *pranayama* by following the same process done during the first round.

Daily Practice: During the first week, do two rounds only. From the second week onwards, do three to four rounds of *Bhastrika pranayama. Never* do more than four rounds in a single day.

Benefits: This *pranayama* is unique in curing respiratory problems. It removes lung troubles and congestion of the nasal passages. It is excellent for removing any heart and chest ailments. It also affects the whole digestive system. It can be practiced by people of any age and sex.

HEADACHE

Of all the diseases prevalent in our society, headache (in one form or another) has become one of the most common problems of our time. It would not be out of place to mention that perhaps no one is spared from this malady. Each of us has experienced a headache of some sort at some time in our lives. In the United States, headaches are so common among office workers that pain-relieving drugs are always kept on hand and some people take a few tablets daily to get rid of their headache.

People suffer from various types of headaches. Some suffer constantly from headaches for years; others have them only now and then. Many others often get a headache at certain times of the day. In certain cases, there is pain in only half of the forehead. Chronic headache is called "migraine." There are various causes for headaches, a comprehensive list of which is not easy to present; but, some of their well-known causes are listed below.

Causes: When the nervous system of an individual is subjected to either internal or external strain and stress, one develops a headache. Because the head is the center of all the nerves, any disorder which affects them consequently begins to show its impact on the central nervous system, resulting in head pain. This straining of the nerves can be caused by high or low blood pressure; gastric trouble; constipation; wind problems; indigestion; sinus; eye pain or trouble; excessive smoking; use of tobacco in any form; excessive intake of coffee, tea, or alcoholic drinks; lack of proper rest and sleep; anxiety; tension; and fatigue. Whatever the cause or causes of headache, it is curable through the yogic method of treatment permanently. Let me describe the yogic way of curing this trouble.

Cure: The yogic method of treatment of headache is comprised of three aspects: (i) avoiding those daily items which strain the nerves; (ii) eating a proper diet; and (iii) practicing some selected *asanas, pranayamas,* and *bandhas.*

Persons suffering from headaches should not drink more than two cups of tea or coffee in a day; should cut down on, or completely stop, smoking or using tobacco in any form. Those alcoholic drinks should be stopped which cause hangovers. Patients should sleep for six to eight hours per day and avoid being tense or angry. They should live in an environment where plenty of fresh air is available. These are some essential precautions which need to be paid due attention to for avoiding this pain.

The diet chart for headache patients is the same as that described in Chapter 2 (under the section "Abdominal Disorders"). It must be added that fruits, green vegetables, salad, and any leafy vegetable should be taken daily, together with other regular food. Patients must not eat fried foods. They should drink ten to fifteen glasses of fresh water every twenty-four hours, should eat lightly, and avoid spices, especially those with a sharp flavor. By taking their diet according to the diet chart of Chapter 2, and by paying attention to the suggestions and recommendations made above, they should practice the following yogic exercises:

Yoga Practice: *Asanas, pranayamas,* and *bandhas* for curing headaches:

(i) *Surya Namaskar asana:* as described in Chapter 2.
(ii) *Bhujanga asana:* as described in Chapter 2.
(iii) *Jalandhar bandha:* as described in Chapter 8.
(iv) *Rechaka-Puraka pranayama:* as described in Chapter 2.
(v) *Shitali pranayama:* as described below.
(vi) *Shava asana:* for five to ten minutes at the end, as described in Chapter 2.

SHITALI PRANAYAMA

Shitali means cooling, and this is a *pranayama* which cools the whole body. In this *pranayama,* air is inhaled through the mouth slowly and constantly, and is exhaled through both nostrils in the same way. This cools the whole body and, at the same time, relaxes the central nervous system. It is an easy *pranayama* which can be done by people of any age.

Position of Readiness: Be seated either in *Padma asana* or *Sukha asana* as shown in Figure 1 or Figure 2. Keep your hands on your knees as shown in Figure 48. Bring your tongue forward to touch the teeth from inside. Open your lips slightly and lift the upper teeth a bit so that there is a gap between the upper and lower teeth for sucking air as shown in Figure 49. Keep your spine and head straight. Close your eyes and be relaxed. This is the position of readiness for *Shitali pranayama.*

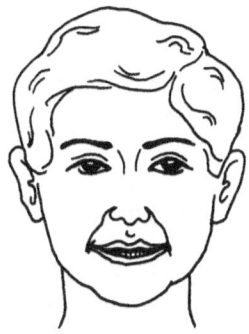

Figure 49. Shitali Pranayama

Steps of Actual Practice: (i) Start inhaling air through the mouth in such a way that air is passed all over the tongue. Take in as much air as you can comfortably.

(ii) Just when the inhaling is over, start exhaling through the nostrils slowly and constantly and expel all the air.

(iii) When exhalation is over, start inhaling through the mouth and between the teeth and exhaling through the nostrils continuously. One inhalation and one exhalation make one round. Do this for ten rounds.

(iv) After doing ten rounds of this *pranayama*, rest for about thirty seconds. While resting, keep your mouth closed and breathe normally. Feel the cooling effect of the *pranayama* in the mouth, throat, head, and all over the body. After resting for the desired period, do ten more rounds in the way as in the first.

Daily Practice: Do twenty to thirty rounds of this *pranayama* daily in units of ten at a time, and rest for thirty seconds after every ten units as described above. It is important that, while resting, you keep your mouth closed and breathe normally. Do not talk while resting. Silence while resting will have a greater effect of cooling the nerves all over the body.

Benefits: It has a great energizing, soothing, relaxing, and cooling effect on all the nerve channels and the whole body. People suffering from high blood pressure, gastric troubles, tension, and anxiety will find this *pranayama* very effective in removing these disorders.

In yogic literature, it is said that if one feels thirsty or hungry in a place where water and food are not available, this *pranayama* satisfies both thirst and hunger. Since it has a great cooling effect on the system, it is just possible that some practitioners may catch cold or get a sore throat by practicing it. If this happens, they are advised to gargle with hot saline water. This gargling with salted water will remove the cold caused by *Shitali*.

CHAPTER 10

Eye Disorders

IN THIS section, the yogic method of curing certain eye defects concerned specifically with the power of vision is described. It must be emphasized that the yogic method of cure is not used to correct organic defects such as cataracts, glaucoma, and other disorders of this nature. These defects must be treated by eye specialists. But in those cases where surgical treatment is not necessary, disorders like eyestrain, eye pain, diminishing vision, near and far sightedness, and other visual defects can be cured through the yogic system. Further, problems like watering of the eyes, itching in the region of the eyes, blurred vision, and redness in one or both eyes can easily be cured through the yogic method. In other words, eye defects which do not require any surgery and are considered curable through medicinal aids can be cured through yoga without the use of any medicines.

Disorders of the eye, especially those affecting visual power, are becoming an alarming problem all over the world. The problem is more acute in the developing countries than in the advanced ones. One primary cause for this is related to malnutrition. We know that millions cannot afford to eat a proper diet which affects the health and, ultimately, the vision. Although an individual may be quite normal and free from disease, due to a lack of proper nourishment, his health and the power of his eyes gradually weaken. Consequently, even when there is no specific disease in the eyes, the vision continues to deteriorate. First let me point out the causes of these eye troubles.

Causes: When everything else is normal but one still develops some eye disorder of a non-organic type, it is mainly due to a faulty diet and certain undesirable habits. For example, many habitually eat mostly fried, highly spiced, and seasoned food. Some develop the habit of drinking excessive amounts of coffee, tea, or hard liquor; smoking excessively; lacking rest or sleep; and unduly straining the eyes. There are three categories of those who suffer in this respect: (i) those who can afford proper food, but are in the habit of eating only a particular type of food which causes malnutrition; (ii) those who are financially unable to afford to eat a balanced diet; and (iii) those who suffer from certain identified undesirable habits. The patients of all three categories can correct their eye defects with only a little attention and care.

Cure: Patients suffering from any visual disorder need to pay special attention to their diets and to correcting certain habits. They *must stop eating* those things which are harmful to the vision, and they *should eat* those things which are conducive to the growth and restoration of the vision.

What Not To Eat

They should not eat fatty, fried, and hard to digest foods; and they should stop eating meat, chicken, and highly seasoned or spicy foods. They should avoid eating pickles, red pepper, and other items which strain the nerves. They should not drink coffee and tea. Use of tobacco in any form and smoking should be stopped.

What To Eat

The main consideration should be on a balanced diet. Having a balanced diet depends more on making an effort than on spending money. It does not cost much to have all the ingredients of a balanced diet. The primary consideration is to include salad, green and leafy vegetables, and fruits of any kind in your daily intake. You should eat according to the diet chart below:

Breakfast (7 to 9 A.M.)

(i)	Any fresh fruit juice	
	or	
	Vegetable or tomato juice	— ½ glass
(ii)	Fresh sweet apple or any fresh fruit	— as desired
(iii)	Cereal, wheat germ, or oatmeal with milk and honey	— as desired
	or	
	Whole wheat bread or English muffin	— one or two slices
(iv)	Sprouted chick-peas	— ¼ cup
(v)	Milk or Ovaltine	— one cup

Lunch and Dinner (12 noon to 2 P.M. and 6 to 8 P.M.)

(i)	Salad (a mixture of lettuce, tomato, cucumber, celery, beets, watercress, radish, carrots, and sprouts) with a little salt and lemon juice, with salad dressing, or plain	— one bowl
(ii)	Vegetable or bean soup	— one cup
(iii)	Wheat bread or rice	— as desired
(iv)	Green vegetables (any kind)	— as desired
(v)	Leafy vegetables (any kind)	— as desired
(vi)	Fish or liver (for non-vegetarians)	— on alternate days
(vii)	Yogurt or buttermilk	— as desired

Afternoon Refreshment (3 to 5 P.M.)

(i)	Fresh fruits (any kind)	— as desired
(ii)	Raw nuts (not fried or roasted)	— as desired
(iii)	Cheese	— one slice
(iv)	Ovaltine with milk or table cream	— one cup if desired

The important point to be kept in mind is that the main course of your daily diet should consist of salad, fresh fruits, and green vegetables. Food should be cooked in vegetable oils with very little or no spices. Special attention should be paid to observing the following principles while eating:

Principles and Requirements of Eating

(i) Eat slowly and chew the food very thoroughly.

(ii) Eat (especially dinner) at least two hours prior to sleeping at night.

(iii) Never eat more than eighty-five percent of your stomach's capacity at any time. In other words, always eat a little less than you need.

(iv) Avoid drinking water while eating. Drink water half an hour after eating, and take ten to fifteen glasses of fresh water every twenty-four hours.

By following the principles and method of eating described above, and by practicing the following yoga *asanas* daily, you can be sure of curing your eye problems.

Yoga Practice:

(i) Surya Namaskar asana: as described in Chapter 3.

(ii) Trikona asana: as described in Chapter 5.

(iii) Bhujanga asana: as described in Chapter 2.

(iv) Yoga mudra: as described in Chapter 4.

(v) Jalandhar bandha: as described in Chapter 8.

(vi) Shava asana: at the end, as described in Chapter 2.

(vii) Eye exercises: as described below.

It is advised to practice these yoga *asanas* in the same order in which they are listed. At the end of the yoga practice, one should rest in *Shava asana* for about five minutes. When the *Shava asana* is over, the eye exercises should be practiced.

EYE EXERCISES

We are going to describe two types of eye exercises. These exercises have been divided into Group "A" and Group "B."

Eye Exercise "A"

In this exercise, you are going to move the eyes without moving the head and neck. You have to keep your head, neck, and spine erect and move only the eyes as directed. Do not pull your eyes excessively in any direction. Make the movement without any excessive strain on the eyes. Try to develop a rhythm in moving the eyes. With this understanding, begin your practice as described below:

(i) Be seated comfortably. Keep the spine, neck, and head straight and in one line. Look directly ahead at eye level. Breathe normally. This is the position of readiness.

(ii) Look up towards the sky or ceiling for two seconds. Then look down towards the earth for two seconds. Again look upwards for two seconds and then downwards for two seconds. Do this upward and downward movement twice. This makes one unit of the exercise. After doing this, close your eyes for two seconds.

(iii) Then open your eyes and look straight ahead. Now look towards the right as far as you can for two seconds. Then look towards the left side and stay there for two seconds while trying to see as far as possible. Look again to the right, then to the left. Now look in front again. Close your eyes. One unit of this left-right exercise is over. Keep your eyes closed for six to eight seconds.

Note: Remember that one unit of up-down movement plus one unit of right-left movement are counted together as one round of this eye exercise. When one round is over, rest for six to eight seconds. After resting for a few seconds, make two more rounds of this up-down and left-right exercise.

Daily Practice: During the first week, do two rounds daily. From the second week onwards, do three to four rounds daily. After doing the desired rounds, do the palming as suggested below:

Palming

Rub your palms against one another so that heat is generated in the palms by friction. After rubbing the palms in this way for six to eight seconds, place the left palm on the left eye and the right palm on the right eye as shown in Figure 50. When you place the palms on the eyes, no pressure should be felt on the eyes. The palms should be pressed lightly on the outer part of the eye region. When the palms cover the eyes, keep them there for eight to ten seconds.

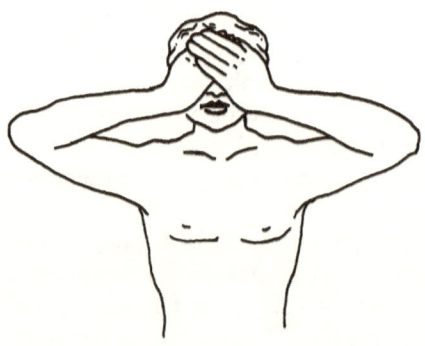

Figure 50. Palming the Eye

After eight to ten seconds, remove the palms and rest. This completes one round of palming. After resting for six to eight seconds, do two more rounds of palming. You can add the following eye exercise of Group "B" from the second week onward.

Eye Exercise "B"

In this exercise you move the eyes in a clockwise and counterclockwise motion. To do this Group "B" exercise, follow the steps described below:

(i) Look straight ahead. Lift your eyes up and start moving them in a circle: coming to the right side and then going down, then to the left side, and then upward again. This makes one unit of clockwise exercise. Repeat this twice and rest for six to eight seconds. While resting, keep your eyes closed.

(ii) Now move the eyes counterclockwise: Look in front of you. Then look up towards the ceiling, then to the left, then downward, then come to the right side, and then upward again in a circular way. This makes one counterclockwise eye movement. Perform this movement twice. Now rest for six to eight seconds. While resting, keep the eyes closed.

One unit of clockwise and one unit of the counterclockwise exercise make one round of this "B" exercise. Do this clockwise and counterclockwise exercise for two rounds and then rest for ten seconds by closing your eyes. After the rest is over, do the palming three to four times. After palming, your exercise is over.

Daily Practice: From the second week onward, first practice four rounds of Group "A." Then do four rounds of Group "B." After completing the exercise of Groups A and B, do four rounds of palming at the end.

These eyes exercises can be practiced twice, independently, within twenty-four hours. This means that you can do only the eye exercises without doing yoga. Those practicing twice should allow a gap of eight hours between sessions.

CHAPTER 11

Heart Ailments
and High Blood Pressure

MILLIONS OF people suffer from diseases of the heart and blood vessels which are called "Cardiovascular Diseases." This type of disorder has become "the number-one killer disease" in developed countries like the United States and Western Europe, and it is increasing rapidly in the developing countries. According to the American Medical Association, more than fifty percent of all deaths in the United States every year are caused by cardiovascular diseases and this type of disease is called "the epidemic of the 20th century."[1]

Therefore, it is very important to know what these cardio-vascular diseases are, what causes them, and how they can be controlled, cured, and prevented through Therapeutic Yoga. Since these diseases are related to the heart and the blood vessels, some basic understanding of these organs is essential.

The heart is a tough muscular organ whose constant function is to pump blood to the arteries at an average rate of 70 to 75

---

[1]See American Medical Association. *Today's Health Guide* (U.S.A.: A.M.A., 1968). p. 380.

times per minute. The heart keeps the blood circulating by receiving it in its chambers from every part of the body through the veins, and then pumping it to all parts of the body through the arteries.

When any part of the circulatory system does not receive the needed blood supply, it is damaged. This damage could be in the heart itself or in the lungs, kidneys, the brain, or other organs. If the heart's mechanism breaks down, a heart ailment, or heart attack, results.

Those diseases associated with the cardiovascular system which can be treated through Therapeutic Yoga are: arteriosclerosis (hardening of the arteries), coronary thrombosis (sudden blockage of the arteries of the heart), degenerative heart diseases, and hypertensive diseases.

Arteriosclerosis: The inner walls of the arteries thicken due to gradual deposits of fatty material. These deposits form layers in the inner walls of the arteries and, as a result, they obstruct the flow of blood. Consequently, blood clots occur in the roughened areas and the blood circulation is blocked.

Coronary Thrombosis: There is a *sudden blocking* of one of the arteries or its branches and the supply of blood to the heart is then partially or wholly affected. The sudden blocking occurs because a clot is deposited in an already narrow artery. Due to the lack of blood supply, a heart attack results. Some symptoms of an attack may be pain in the chest and arms and, sometimes, perspiration.

Degenerative Heart Disease: It occurs because of the gradual decay of the blood vessels. It is thought that excessive tobacco smoking causes this degeneration.[2] The disease generally occurs among middle-aged and elderly persons. In this case,

---

[2]See Dr. Alice Chase, *Nutrition for Health* (New York, Parker Publishing Company, 1967), p. 68.

although the heart muscle continues to work, it is not strong enough to function normally.

Hypertensive Heart Disease: This ailment is a result of the constant presence of high blood pressure in an individual. When the blood pressure continues to remain very high, it overstrains the heart muscle and the whole circulatory system. This overstraining causes wear and tear on the tissues, leads to the hardening of the blood vessels, and reduces the supply of blood to the heart and brain. Sometimes the supply of blood to the brain is so diminished that one or both sides of the body may become paralyzed.

It is now commonly accepted that psychosomatic factors are a major cause of cardiovascular ailments. The illness resulting from strain and stress is known as a "psychosomatic" one (the word being comprised of two Greek words, *psyche* and *soma*, which mean mind and body).

The most common strains and stresses are due to nervousness, which is caused by fear, anxiety, apprehension, tension, and restlessness; anger; jealousy; frustration; depression; and other similar feelings.

In yoga, it is held that the mind controls, governs, and activates the body. In this sense, the body becomes a tool of the mind. What happens is that the mind-straining factors also begin to strain the body's systems. Most modern diseases such as heart ailments, hypertension, asthma, and others are mostly related to these mental strains and stresses which are called, in medical terms, "psychosomatic factors."

Since this chapter covers both heart ailments and high blood pressure, it would be proper to describe the latter briefly before recommending yogic treatment.

High Blood Pressure

In a normal, healthy person the blood pressure remains 120 systolic and 80 diastolic. But when there are abnormalities in the arteries or in the circulatory system, the systolic pressure rises very high and, at times, the diastolic also rises.

This rise in pressure is caused by the narrowness of the arteries, and the heart has to work harder to push the blood through them, resulting in high blood pressure, or hypertension.

Though it is normal for the blood pressure to rise during excitement and at certain emotional moments, it goes down shortly afterward. Such fluctuations do not cause any harmful effects. But when the blood pressure continues to remain excessively high, it causes various disorders such as weakness, fatigue, headache, and, at times, difficulty in breathing, ill temper, vision problems, and a lack of circulation in the extremities.

It is a medically established fact that hypertension may at times be caused by psychosomatic factors. It could also be due to advancing age and its degenerative factors. In the following pages, the process of treating hypertension, as well as heart ailments, is described.

Yogic Process of Treatment

It must be emphasized that Therapeutic Yoga is not a treatment for an emergency case of heart attack or severe hypertension. Therapeutic Yoga should be practiced when the individual concerned is not affected by any type of emergency.

In our treatment at the Indian Institute of Yoga, Patna, we have found that patients with heart ailments regained their normal health within two to three months of yoga practice. Further, once the health was restored, the patients remained in good health without any complaints. Likewise, in cases of high blood pressure, we have found that the circulatory system normalized within one to two months when the patient followed our instructions.

It is significant to mention that the yoga system of treatment is the same for heart ailments and for hypertension. It is comprised of three steps: (i) observing certain principles and advices, (ii) eating a proper diet, and (iii) practicing yoga on a selected basis.

Principles and Advices: Patients with both ailments should stop smoking cigarettes and using tobacco in any form, and should give up tea, coffee, and alcoholic drinks. The intake of butter, cream, eggs, meat, and food containing excessive fat should be stopped.

Hot spices, pickles, chutney, red chili, and the excessive use of salt should be excluded from the diet, and patients must avoid overeating at all times. They must stop working late hours and rest longer during the night.

For a detailed understanding about diet, bathing, cleaning, and other yogic principles, users of this section are advised to read Chapter 1 of this book thoroughly. Some important advices which are not covered in that chapter are mentioned below:

One major recommendation is to relax and keep yourself free from anxiety, nervousness, tension, and restlessness. Though it is not easy for everyone to be relaxed in every condition and situation, it can be done with a proper understanding of the **Self, Society,** and **Nature.** These aspects are discussed in Chapter 7 and you are advised to read it carefully to develop the self-power for overcoming these tension-creating problems.[3] You should eat according the diet chart given below:

Breakfast (7 to 9 A.M.)

(i) Any fresh juice or vegetable juice	— ½ glass
(ii) Papaya, fresh apple, or other fruits	— as desired
(iii) Chick-pea sprouts	— one handful
(iv) Whole wheat bread (without butter)	— one or two
or	slices
Wheat germ with skim milk	— one cup
(v) Skim milk (if desired)	— one cup

---

[3]Those interested in further reading are advised to see Dr. Phulgenda Sinha, *Yoga: Meaning, Values and Practice* (Patna, Indian Institute of Yoga, 1970), pp. 32-72.

Lunch and Dinner (12 noon to 2 P.M. and 6 to 8 P.M.)

(i) Salad (a mixture of carrot, lettuce, watercress, beets, cucumber, tomato, celery, radish, and bean sprouts) with a little salt and lemon juice or plain, or with salad dressing	— one medium bowl
(ii) Vegetable or bean soup	— one cup
(iii) Whole wheat bread (without butter) or rice	— as desired
(iv) Fresh green vegetables (stewed or boiled)	— as desired
(v) Fresh leafy vegetables (steamed)	— as desired
(vi) Fish (broiled) for non-vegetarians	— one or two moderate pieces on alternate days
(vii) Non-fat yogurt or buttermilk	— one cup, if desired

Afternoon Refreshment (3 to 5 P.M.)

(i) Fresh fruits (any kind)	— as desired
(ii) Fresh green peas (boiled)	— as desired
(iii) Ovaltine or herb tea with milk	— one cup, if desired

The important points to be kept in mind are that a major part of the daily diet should be of salad, fresh fruits, and green vegetables; and dishes should be cooked in vegetable oils and with little or no spices.

Yoga Practice: Patients with heart ailments and hypertension should practice yoga in phases, according to the guidelines given below:

First Phase: In this phase, which should last for three weeks, only *Shava asana* needs to be practiced. A detailed description about the method of practicing *Shava asana* is given in Chapter 2. Practitioners should first read and properly understand the process of *Shava asana* bfore actually doing it. One important advice is to not practice it in a hurry. Do it thoroughly and patiently. Be at ease when you practice *Shava asana*.

Daily Practice: *Shava asana* should be done twice or three times daily. At one stretch, it should be performed for about thirty to forty minutes. The most suitable times for practicing it are in the morning (before breakfast), in the afternoon (two hours after lunch), and in the evening. The main consideration is that the stomach should be empty while practicing *Shava asana*.

Those suffering from high blood pressure should be examined by a doctor to find out their condition after practicing *Shava asana* for three weeks. By this time, the blood pressure should definitely be normalized. When the pressure becomes normal, patients should add the *asanas* of the second and third phases described below. But if the blood pressure remains above 150 systolic, they should keep practicing only *Shava asana* until the pressure is normal.

Benefits: Although the benefits of *Shava asana* have already been mentioned in Chapter 2, a few words need to be added here. Our experience shows that a regular and proper practice of *Shava asana* for about two to three weeks has a remarkably good effect on patients with heart ailments and high blood pressure. It corrects disorders of the circulatory system by relaxing the nerves and the internal organs. Because the arteries are normalized and relaxed, the high blood pressure is reduced and is gradually corrected.

Second Phase (Fourth and Fifth Weeks): Before practicing yoga in this phase, the practitioner must read "Essentials of Yoga Practice" as described in Chapter 1, with special attention to the rest requirements. After practicing *Shava asana* twice or three times daily during the First Phase, the following *asanas* should be added and the practice should be in the numerical order listed below:

(i) *Pawana Mukta asana* (in the lying position): This *asana* is comprehensively described in Chapter 2. Practice it without straining yourself; do only as much as you can comfortably. Make four to six rounds daily.

(ii) *Uttanapada asana* (with only one leg at a time): It is fully described in Chapter 2. In the beginning, hold the leg up for only a few seconds. Gradually increase the time to four seconds, then to six. Daily practice should be only six rounds (three rounds with each leg).

(iii) *Shava asana:* When other *asanas* are practiced, *Shava asana* should be done at the end. The method of practicing *Shava asana* is the same as during the first phase. The duration of *Shava asana*, when done after yoga practice, may be reduced, if so desired. A practice of fifteen to thirty minutes should be sufficient.

During this second phase, *Shava asana* should continue to be practiced singly also, at least one more time during a period of twenty-four hours.

Third Phase (Sixth Week and Afterward): During this phase and afterward, the daily practice of yoga should be in the following order:

(*i*) *Pranayama* (with *Rechaka* and *Puraka*): Its method of practice is well illustrated and described in Chapter 2. Practice according to the directions given there.

(*ii*) *Surya Namaskar asana:* as described in Chapter 3.

(*iii*) *Santulan asana:* as described in Chapter 5.

(*iv*) *Pawana Mukta asana:* as done in Phase Two.

(*v*) *Uttanapada asana:* as done in Phase Two.

(*vi*) *Shava asana:* Practice of this *asana* should be for a minimum of fifteen minutes.

CHAPTER 12

Prevention and Control of Alcoholism and Drug Abuse

SINCE IT has been well established that the destructive power of alcohol and drugs is more or less the same, the process of preventing and overcoming addiction to both is comprehensively described in this chapter. When one becomes addicted to alcohol or drugs, the individual feels helpless about giving up the habit and his health can degenerate to the point of a premature death. The yogic process for preventing the use of alcohol and drugs, rehabilitating damaged health, and developing self-discipline and control is the same in both cases. For this reason, I prefer to discuss them together in this section.

Although there have been serious efforts by various social and governmental agencies to help prevent addiction, it has been found that drug use by young people in the United States has rapidly increased since the 1960's. In a survey conducted by the National Institute of Drug Abuse in 1979, it was found that 65 percent of the 1979 high-school seniors had tried drugs and alcohol; over 10 percent used marijuana daily; 7 percent drank alcohol daily; 25 percent smoked cigarettes daily; and over one-third had used drugs more potent than marijuana such as stimulants, inhalants, and hallucinogens.[1]

According to the *1978 Third Special Report to the U.S. Congress on Alcohol and Health*, 7 percent (9.3 to 10 million) of the 145 million adults in the United States are problem drinkers.[2]

It has also been found that alcohol-related deaths could be as high as 205,000 per year in the United States (11 percent of the 1.9 million deaths in 1975). Clinical studies have shown that alcohol problems in males are associated with mortality rates two to six times higher than rates in the general population.[3]

The consequences of alcoholism and drug abuse are well known and need not be listed here. However, it must be pointed out that heart disease, cancer, hypertension, liver damage, serious nervous and mental disorders, and permanent brain damage are some of the most frightening results of heavy drinking and the use of drugs in various forms.[4] In addition to physical and mental damage, the use of alcohol and drugs shortens the life span, destroys the family and social relationships, and makes mere existence miserable.

The problem of drug abuse and alcoholism is not confined to any particular nation or area. It is becoming a worldwide issue of great public concern. There was a time when alcohol and drugs were taken by a very limited number of people, especially adults, in certain areas and of certain classes. But in recent years, the use of drugs by young people and alcohol consumption by all groups around the world have increased greatly.

There are three facets of the problem: (i) how to prevent

---

[1]*Straight Talk on Drugs* (a publication by Drug Fair, Inc., with the National Institute of Drug Abuse), 1980.

[2]*Third Special Report to the U.S. Congress on Alcohol and Health* (U.S. Department of Health, Education and Welfare), 1978, p. XI.

[3]Ibid.

[4]For details on the harmful effects of drugs and alcohol, see *What Parents Should Know About Drugs* (a publication of Drug Fair, Inc., with the National Institute of Drug Abuse), 1980.

alcohol and drug addiction, (ii) how to restore normal life to those who are already addicted, and (iii) how to rehabilitate and correct the lost or damaged health of the long-time addict. The process of helping those in all three categories through yoga is described in the following pages.

ADDICTION PREVENTION

Prevention of alcohol and drug abuse is easier than rescuing the addicted person. With only a little effort, the lives of millions can be saved through the practice of Hatha Yoga, Seeded Meditation, and with some knowledge of the basic principles, theories, and philosophy of Yoga Science. This observation is based on my personal experience of teaching yoga to more than 20,000 people of various ages, different nationalities, and of mixed socioeconomic and cultural backgrounds.

Among those whom I have taught, there must be hundreds whom I have known and watched closely over a number of years. Though many of them take an occasional social drink, none is alcoholic. Similarly, I have not seen any yoga practitioner using drugs of any kind.

There is a reason why yoga practitioners are not addicted to either drugs or alcohol. Yoga, when practiced even for fifteen minutes daily, creates a power of resistance, develops self-discipline, control, strong inner conviction, and a harmonious physical and mental state. As a result, the stress and strain of modern-day society do not cause anxiety, tension, or nervousness in yoga practitioners. Being free from tension, the probability of taking drugs or alcohol is, hence, greatly reduced.

Why does someone become addicted to drugs or alcohol? It is primarily because the individual uses them to evade, forget, or suppress the anxiety-causing conditions of life. The regular use of alcohol and drugs becomes a habit and, when the same pattern continues, addiction results.

Unfortunately, the youths of today, living in industrial societies, are increasingly faced with anxiety, stress, and strain to the same degree as adults. There is little wonder, then, that youths try to escape these situations by using alcohol, drugs, or tobacco as adults do.

Keeping these aspects of life in mind, it would appear proper to recommend a routine of daily yoga practice for youths and adults alike to prevent those conditions faced by compulsive users of drugs or alcohol.

Recommendations: (i) Young people should be taught the practices and principles of Yoga Science from their high-school days onward. A regular practice of even fifteen minutes daily will greatly reduce the tendency to use drugs, alcohol, and tobacco.

(ii) Adults who are not addicted to alcohol or drugs would find a fifteen minute yoga practice sufficient for maintaining good health and, at the same time, would acquire a built-in power to resist addiction to any harmful substance.

(iii) A chart of daily yoga practice is given separately in the last section of this book. Readers are advised to follow the guidelines mentioned there and to select the *asanas* of daily practice suited to their physical capabilities.

CONTROLLING ADDICTION

By following the yogic process, addiction to drugs or alcohol can be controlled and overcome. While treating a few cases of drug and alcohol addiction at the Indian Institute of Yoga, Patna, India, and at the Yoga and Meditation Center, Ibiza, Spain, I found that it takes addicts about two months to break the habit and create a new life pattern.

The above observation is based on the treatment of about one dozen cases of chronic alcoholics and drug addicts. However, further research is needed to establish a more comprehensive process of rehabilitation, especially for those addicts suffering from multiple physical-mental ailments. I am confident that the Yoga System would prove to be less expensive and better than the clinical method for helping people overcome addiction.

The yogic process of treatment is comprised of the following steps: (i) proper diet; (ii) practice of selected *asanas*, *pranayamas,* and *bandhas;* (iii) Seeded Meditation; and (iv) personal counseling based on yogic principles, theories, and philosophy.

Proper Diet: As mentioned in the preceding section of this book, diet affects both the physical and mental conditions of the individual. According to yogic principles, the type of food an individual eats in due time begins to affect the pattern of his thinking, behavior, and personality. Therefore, eating a proper diet should be the first step in correcting addiction.

Before mentioning a diet chart for addicts, let me first point out what they should not eat. Red pepper, chili, garlic, onions, and hot and sharp spices should be avoided; they should not eat fried or highly seasoned food. Though it is not necessary to be a vegetarian, meat, chicken, fish, or seafood of any kind should be avoided or taken in small amounts for two months. They should eat according to the diet chart given below:

Breakfast (7 to 9 A.M.)

(i)	Orange juice or any fresh fruit juice	— ½ glass
(ii)	Fresh sweet apple or any fresh fruit	— as much as you like
(iii)	Sprouted chick-peas	— one handful
(iv)	Corn flakes, oatmeal, or wheat germ with milk and honey	— as desired
	or	
	Whole wheat bread or English muffin	— one or two slices, as desired
(v)	Coffee, tea, herb tea, or Ovaltine	— one cup, if necessary

Lunch and Dinner (12 noon to 2 P.M. and 6 to 8 P.M.)

(i)	Salad (a mixture of lettuce, tomato, watercress, celery, beets, radish, cucumber, spinach) with any kind of salad dressing	— one small bowl
(ii)	Vegetable, bean, or tomato soup	— one cup
(iii)	Wheat bread and rice	— as desired
(iv)	Leafy vegetables (spinach, broccoli, turnip greens, kale)	— as desired
(v)	Fresh vegetables of any kind	— as desired
(vi)	Fish or liver (once a week)	— moderate amount
(vii)	Dessert (pudding, pie, or cake)	— only once a day

Afternoon Refreshment (3 to 4 P.M.)

(i)	Fresh fruits (other than taken during breakfast)	— as much as desired
(ii)	Raw nuts (a mixture of cashews, pecans, almonds, walnuts, pistachios)	— one handful
(iii)	Cheese (any kind)	— one slice
(iv)	Coffee, tea, herb tea, or Ovaltine	— one cup, if necessary

Selected *Asanas* and *Pranayama*

To practice yoga properly, it is important to first understand its "Essentials" as described in Chapter 1 of this book. The benefit of yoga is enhanced many times when done according to certain requirements. Users of this section are therefore advised to read Chapter 1 once or twice before beginning the practice described below:

First Week of Practice:

> (*i*) *Pawana Mukta asana:* six rounds daily, as described in Chapter 2.
>
> (*ii*) *Surya Namaskar asana:* four rounds, as described in Chapter 3.
>
> (*iii*) *Uttanapada asana:* begin with one leg at a time, make six rounds alternately, as described in Chapter 2.
>
> (*iv*) *Shava asana:* for five minutes, as described in Chapter 2.

Second Week of Practice: Keep practicing all the *asanas* of the first week and add the following ones during the second week:

> (*v*) *Bhujanga asana:* four rounds daily, as described in Chapter 2.
>
> (*vi*) *Shalabha asana:* four rounds daily, as described in Chapter 2.

Note: Practice *Shava asana* for seven minutes at the end of all the *asanas*.

Third Week of Practice: Practice the following *asanas*, *pranayama*, and *bandha* in the order they are listed:

> (*i*) *Pawana Mukta asana*
>
> (*ii*) *Surya Namaskar asana*
>
> (*iii*) *Uttanapada asana*
>
> (*iv*) *Bhujanga asana*
>
> (*v*) *Shalabha asana*
>
> (*vi*) *Bhastrika pranayama:* two rounds only during this week and increase to three rounds during the following week; described in Chapter 9.
>
> (*vii*) *Jalandhar bandha:* four rounds daily, as described in Chapter 8.
>
> (*viii*) *Shava asana:* ten to fifteen minutes at the end of all *asanas*.

From the fourth week onward, you might add any other *asana* described in this book into your list of daily practice.

Personal Counseling: (*i*) If you are working, take leave for a week in order to start your yoga practice and begin your diet according to the above-mentioned chart.

(*ii*) Avoid meeting people, especially addicts, for two to three weeks.

(*iii*) Do not go to parties or get-togethers where alcohol or drugs might be served.

(*iv*) When you begin yoga practice and follow the prescribed diet, you might feel body pain, headache, dullness, irritation, or sleepiness for a few days. These symptoms will vanish automatically after three to four days of continued practice.

(*v*) Practice yoga at the same time every day. In case, for some unavoidable reason, you fail to practice on a particular day, continue your practice from the next day. Missing one day in a week is not undesirable.

(*vi*) For learning Seeded Meditation and for acquiring knowledge of yogic principles, theories, and philosophy, the following books written by the author are recommended:

> *Yoga for Mental Power*—explains and teaches Seeded Meditation,
>
> *Yoga for Total Living*—describes yogic philosophy and theories.

Both books are published by: Orient Paperbacks, 36 C, Connaught Place, New Delhi, India.

Yoga Practice for
Maintaining Good Health

Since the publication of *Yogic Cure for Common Diseases* in 1976, I have received numerous letters of appreciation from every part of India and from other countries. A great number of patients who have been cured from their chronic diseases through this book have requested me to suggest yoga *asanas* they should practice daily to maintain good health and to prevent the recurrence of their disorders. In accordance with those requests, a chart of yoga practice is presented here.

The chart is so made that it will benefit those practitioners who have been cured from certain disorders, as well as those who wish to practice yoga for physical fitness. Practitioners will have two distinct benefits by performing the *asanas* of this chart: (i) it will prevent a recurrence of the disorders they had suffered from, and (ii) a regular yoga practice will keep them in sound physical and mental health.

Chart: Daily Yoga Practice

In this chart, the *asanas* and *pranayamas* have been divided into several groups according to their nature and bodily impact. Practitioners should select one or two *asanas* from each group according to their preference. The *asanas* from Group I to V are easy and can be performed by persons of any age and in any physical condition. The *asanas* of Group VI are a little difficult and it may not be possible for everyone to practice them. It is advised that those who cannot do the *asanas* in Group VI should select *asanas* from another group and they would still benefit from them. The practice of yoga should be made on the basis of personal convenience, suitability of time, and the condition of the practitioner's body. A regular practice of fifteen minutes per day or at least five days in a week will produce excellent results.

A special advice is that, when you practice yoga even for ten or fifteen minutes, you must do *Shava asana* at the end. For the details of *Shava asana*, see Chapters 1 and 2. Those who would like to practice the eye exercises, concentration, and meditation should do them after the *Shava asana*. Practitioners are advised to see the respective figures and pages of their selected *asanas* for practicing them correctly.

With these clarifications, the chart is listed below:

Group I

Surya Namaskar asana:	two to four rounds; see Chapter 3.
Santulan asana:	two to four rounds; see Chapter 5.
Pawana Mukta asana:	four rounds; see Chapter 2.

Group II

Ujjayee pranayama:	five rounds in the standing or in the lying position; see Chapter 4.
Rechaka-Puraka pranayama:	ten rounds as described in Chapter 2.

Bhastrika pranayama:	ten rounds as described in Chapter 9.

Group III

Trikona asana:	four rounds; see Chapter 5.
Tara asana:	two to four rounds; see Chapter 4.
Ardha Vakra asana	two to four rounds; see Chapter 3.

Group IV

Bhujanga asana:	two to four rounds; see Chapter 2.
Shalabha asana:	two to four rounds to be practiced after *Bhujanga asana;* see Chapter 2.
Pashchimottan asana:	two to four rounds; see Chapter 2.
Uttanapada asana:	two to four rounds; see Chapter 2.
Ekpada Utthan asana:	two to four rounds; see Chapter 4.

Group V

Veera asana:	four rounds; see Chapter 5.
Vriksha asana:	four rounds; see Chapter 5.
Gomukha asana:	four rounds; see Chapter 5.
Yoga mudra:	two to four rounds; see Chapter 4.

Group VI

Sarvanga asana:	one to three minutes; see Chapter 4.
Matsya asana:	two rounds, to be practiced after *Sarvanga asana;* see Chapter 4.
Hala asana:	two to four rounds; see Chapter 7.
Dhanur asana:	two to four rounds; see Chapter 3.

General

Shava asana:	for one-fourth of yoga practicing time (at the end), see Chapter 2.
Eye Exercises:	see Chapter 10.
Concentration and Meditation (if desired):	see Chapter 7.

Selected Bibliography

Early Period

Gherand Samhita
Goraksha Paddhati
Hatha Pradipika
Samkhya Darshan by Kapil
Vasistha Samhitā
Yoga Sutra by Patanjali

Modern Period

Acharya Bhadrasen, *Yoga Aur Swasthya* (Ajmer: Adarsha Sahitya Niketan, 1951).

Swami Kuvalayananda, *Pranayama* (Bombay: Popular Prakashan, 1972).

Swami Kuvalayananda, *Yogasana* (Bombay: Popular Prakashan, 1965).

Dr. Phulgenda Sinha, *Yoga: Meaning, Values and Practice* (Patna: Indian Institute of Yoga, 1970).

Swami Sivananda, *Yoga Asanas* (India: The Divine Life Society, 1972).

Swami Sivananda, *Thought Power* (India: The Divine Life Society, 1970).

Swami Vivekananda, *Jnana Yoga* (India: Ramakrishna Mission).

Swami Vivekananda, *Karma Yoga* (India: Ramakrishna Mission).

Swami Vivekananda, *Raja Yoga* (India: Ramakrishna Mission).

YOGA PRACTICE: WEEKLY REPORT

1st Week Date	Yoga Asanas, Pranayama	How many times?	Food Eaten	Remarks
1st Day				
2nd Day				
3rd Day				
4th Day				
5th Day				
6th Day				
7th Day				

Evaluate progress at the end of week:

YOGA PRACTICE: WEEKLY REPORT

2nd Week Date	Yoga Asanas, Pranayama	How many times?	Food Eaten	Remarks
1st Day				
2nd Day				
3rd Day				
4th Day				
5th Day				
6th Day				
7th Day				

Evaluate progress at the end of 2nd week:

YOGA PRACTICE: WEEKLY REPORT

3rd Week Date	Yoga Asanas, Pranayama	How many times?	Food Eaten	Remarks
1st Day				
2nd Day				
3rd Day				
4th Day				
5th Day				
6th Day				
7th Day				

Evaluate progress at the end of 3rd week:

YOGA PRACTICE: WEEKLY REPORT

4th Week Date	Yoga Asanas, Pranayama	How many times?	Food Eaten	Remarks
1st Day				
2nd Day				
3rd Day				
4th Day				
5th Day				
6th Day				
7th Day				

Evaluate progress at the end of 4th week:

YOGA PRACTICE: WEEKLY REPORT

5th Week Date	Yoga Asanas, Pranayama	How many times?	Food Eaten	Remarks
1st Day				
2nd Day				
3rd Day				
4th Day				
5th Day				
6th Day				
7th Day				

Evaluate progress at the end of 5th week:

YOGA PRACTICE: WEEKLY REPORT

6th Week Date	Yoga Asanas, Pranayama	How many times?	Food Eaten	Remarks
1st Day				
2nd Day				
3rd Day				
4th Day				
5th Day				
6th Day				
7th Day				

Evaluate progress at the end of 6th week:

YOGA PRACTICE: WEEKLY REPORT

7th Week Date	Yoga Asanas, Pranayama	How many times?	Food Eaten	Remarks
1st Day				
2nd Day				
3rd Day				
4th Day				
5th Day				
6th Day				
7th Day				

Evaluate progress at the end of 7th week:

GENERAL NOTES & OBSERVATIONS
at the end of 8th week

About the Author

Phulgenda Sinha is an internationally recognized expert on yoga science, especially the practical treatment of health problems using yoga. He has consulted for the World Health Organization (WHO), the National Institutes of Health (NIH), and the District of Columbia Dept. of Human Services. Other works by Dr. Sinha are: *Yoga—Meaning, Values and Practice, Yogic Cure for Common Diseases, Seeded Meditation, Yoga for Mental Power, Introduction to Yoga Science, Yoga for Total Living, Yog Dwara Rogoan Ki Chikitsa, The Gita as it Was, Yog Sachitra Vijnana, Yoga Sutra of Pantanjali, Samkhya Karika of Kapila, and Dharana Healing.*

978-0-595-36154-0
0-595-36154-4